DENTIST AND PATIENT

Dental procedures explained to the patient

Michele Cassetta

With the collaboration of Carlo Montemezzo

edra
PUBLISHING

Original title
ODONTOIATRA E PAZIENTE – Gli interventi odontoiatrici spiegati al paziente

ISBN: 978-88-214-5067-9

Editor: **Paola Sammaritano**, Edra S.p.a.
Project Manager: **Sandra A. Calarota**, Edra S.p.A.
Paper, Printing and Binding Manager: **Paolo Ficicchia**, Edra S.p.A.
Graphic design: **Tommaso Torelli** - TTDesign

This edition first published 2024

ISBN: 978-1-957260-65-5

edra
PUBLISHING

Edra Publishing US LLC
3309 Northlake Boulevard,
Suite 203, Palm Beach Gardens,
FL, 33403
EIN: 844113980

info@edrapublishing.com
www.edrapublishing.com

Printed in Italy in February 2024 by "Erregiemme printing" S.r.l.

THE AUTHORS

MICHELE CASSETTA

Graduated in Medicine and Surgery, he practices dentistry in Bologna.
Former professor of "Doctor-Patient Communication" at the Faculty of Medicine and Surgery of the University of Bologna. Member of the Strategic Communication Area of the National Federation of Orders of Surgeons and Dentists. Speaker at courses and conferences, he is invited as a speaker and chairman in numerous cultural and informational events. A scientific journalist, author of books and podcasts, he hosts radio and television broadcasts of health information. He writes and performs plays on neuroscience ("*La Mente Latente*"), which he brings to the stage with the jazz musician Gianluca Petrella.

CARLO MONTEMEZZO

Graduated in Communication Sciences at the University of Bologna, with a thesis in sociology of communication involving the Community of San Patrignano, with which he established a solid relationship of collaboration from a human and professional point of view.
Graduated with honors in Dental Hygiene at the University of Ferrara, with a thesis in neurology entitled "Music, anxiety and depression on the perception of pain during professional oral hygiene", in which he explores the relationship between the musical field, which he has always been passionate about, and the dental field. He earned his degree in Dentistry from the Univeristy of Ferrara. He currently practices as a dentist at his family clinic in Ferrara and is a consultant at various clinics in Emilia Romagna.

PREFACE

Carrying out the dental practice requires many skills in addition to the strictly clinical ones that are learned through university studies.

The dentist is called upon to acquire mainly communication notions as it is essential that the patient understands the therapeutic pathways and the nature of the services.

Only in this way can the indispensable therapeutic alliance be born.

In communication, only the outcome matters and never the intention, and verifying the message is a step that is too often underestimated.

We are increasingly confronted with informed patients, and this scenario leads us to behaviors that are not always effective from a communication perspective.

This book aims to be a valid aid both for clinician and patient, contributing substantially to creating and consolidating the basis for a relationship of mutual trust that starts from an interactive, simple but timely explanation of the specific performance.

We know a good deal of the world around us through sight, and the figures stimulate precisely this sense, with the aim of making the patient visualize the nature of the services in a simple and schematic way, offering the dentist the additional possibility of intervening graphically, thanks to the attached marker, to enrich the explanations.

This communication method will have positive repercussions on the acceptance of treatment plans, the creation of a true therapeutic alliance and, last but not least, will serve to keep away possible medico-legal litigations, often generated by the lack of understanding of the therapies.

The description of the intervention thus becomes the intervention of the description, essential for making the patient truly aware and the clinician truly competent.

Good use and good work!

Michele Cassetta, Carlo Montemezzo

TABLE OF CONTENTS

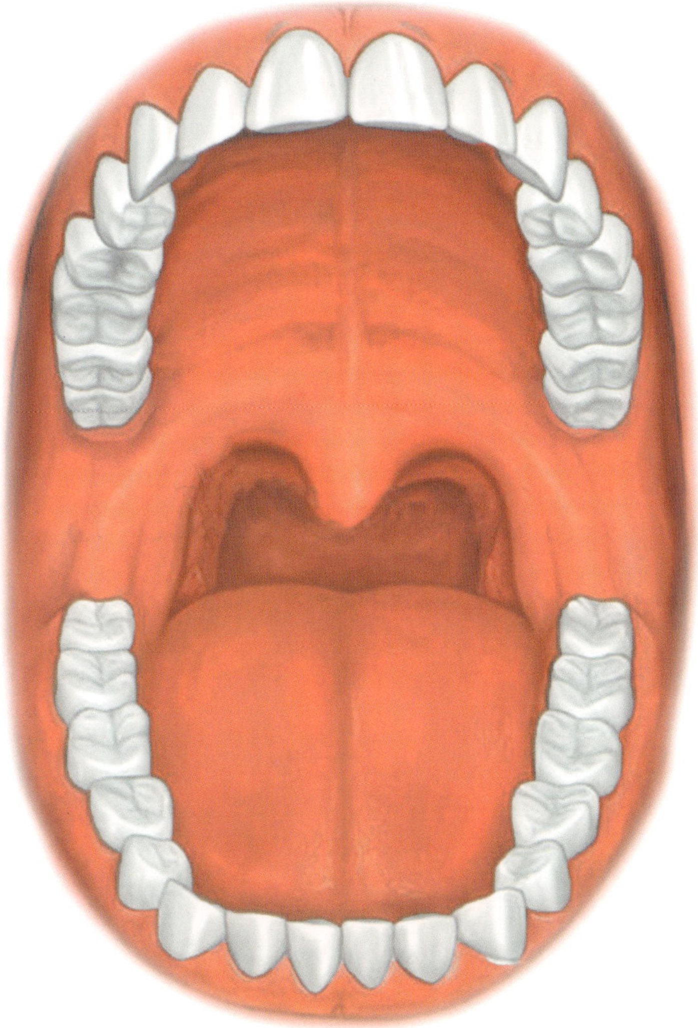

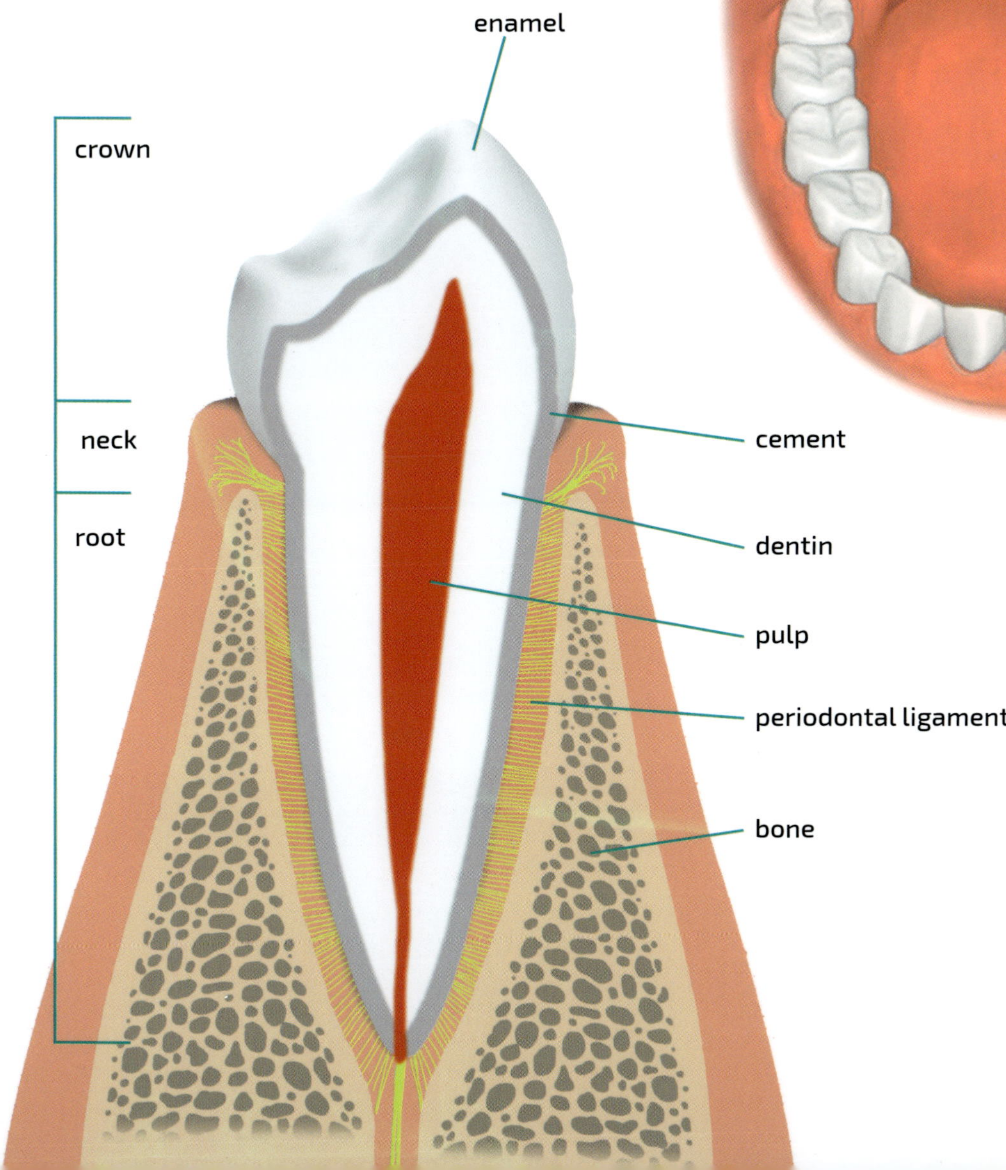
enamel
crown
neck
root
cement
dentin
pulp
periodontal ligament
bone

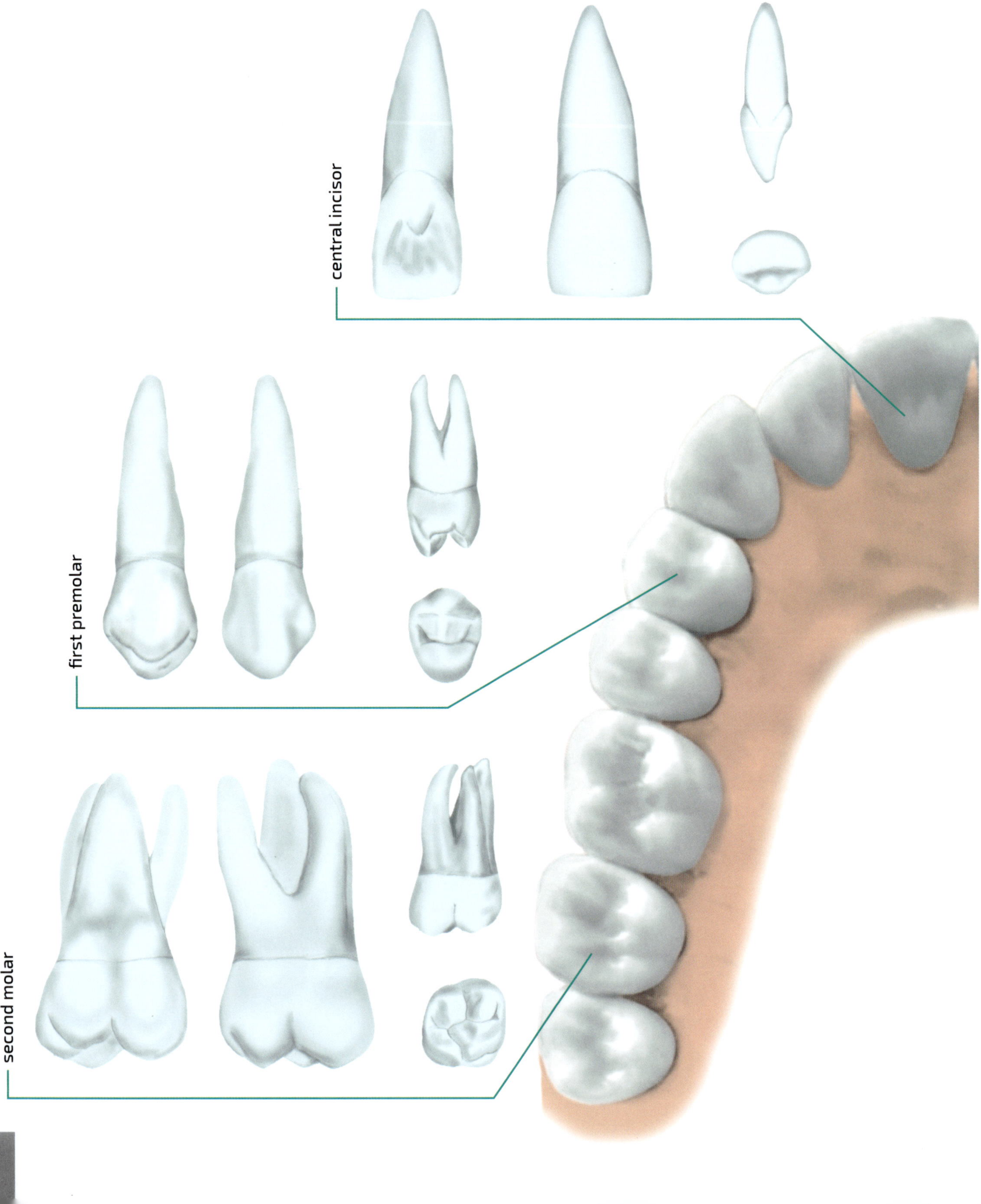
central incisor
first premolar
second molar

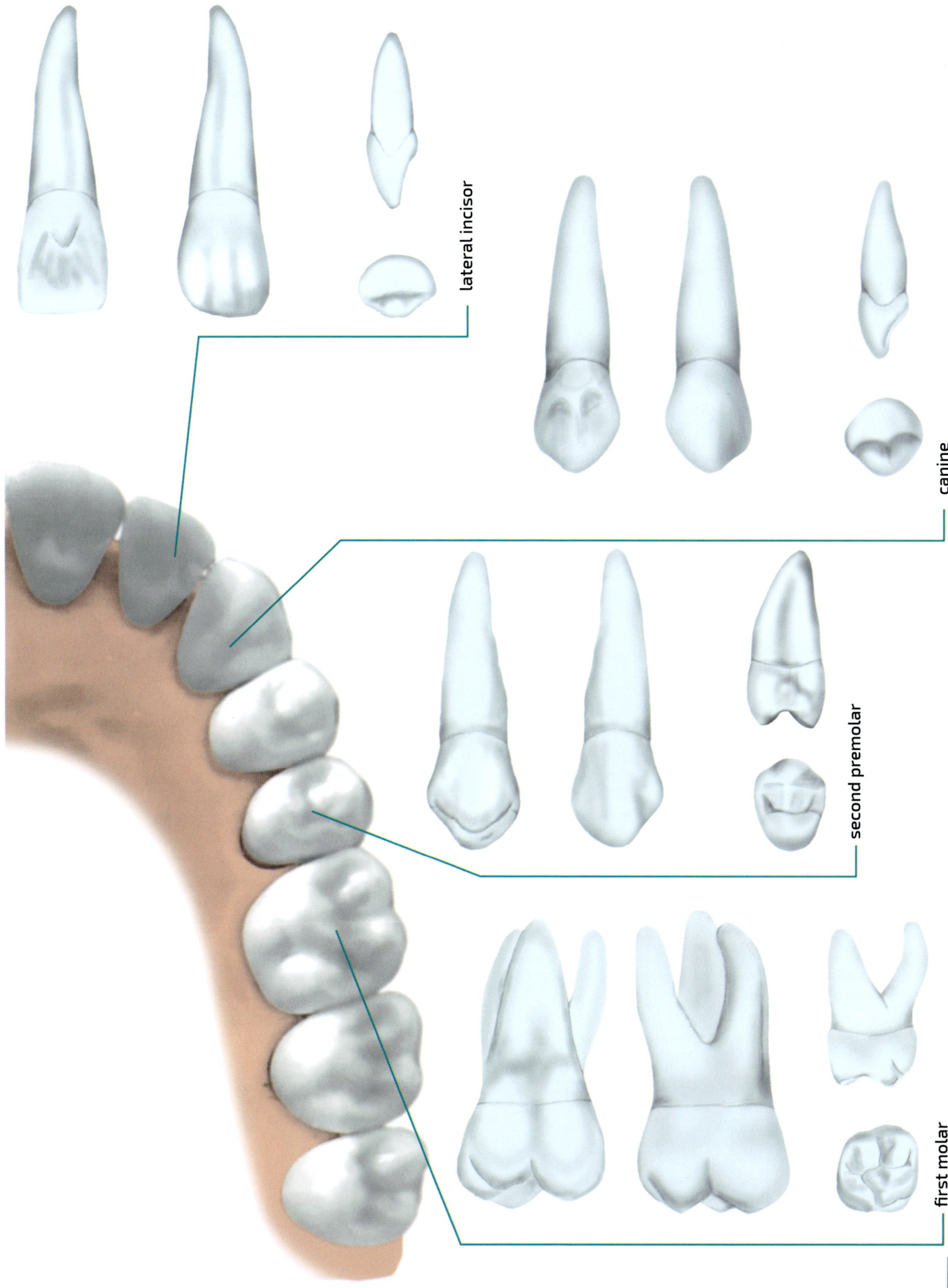
lateral incisor
canine
second premolar
first molar

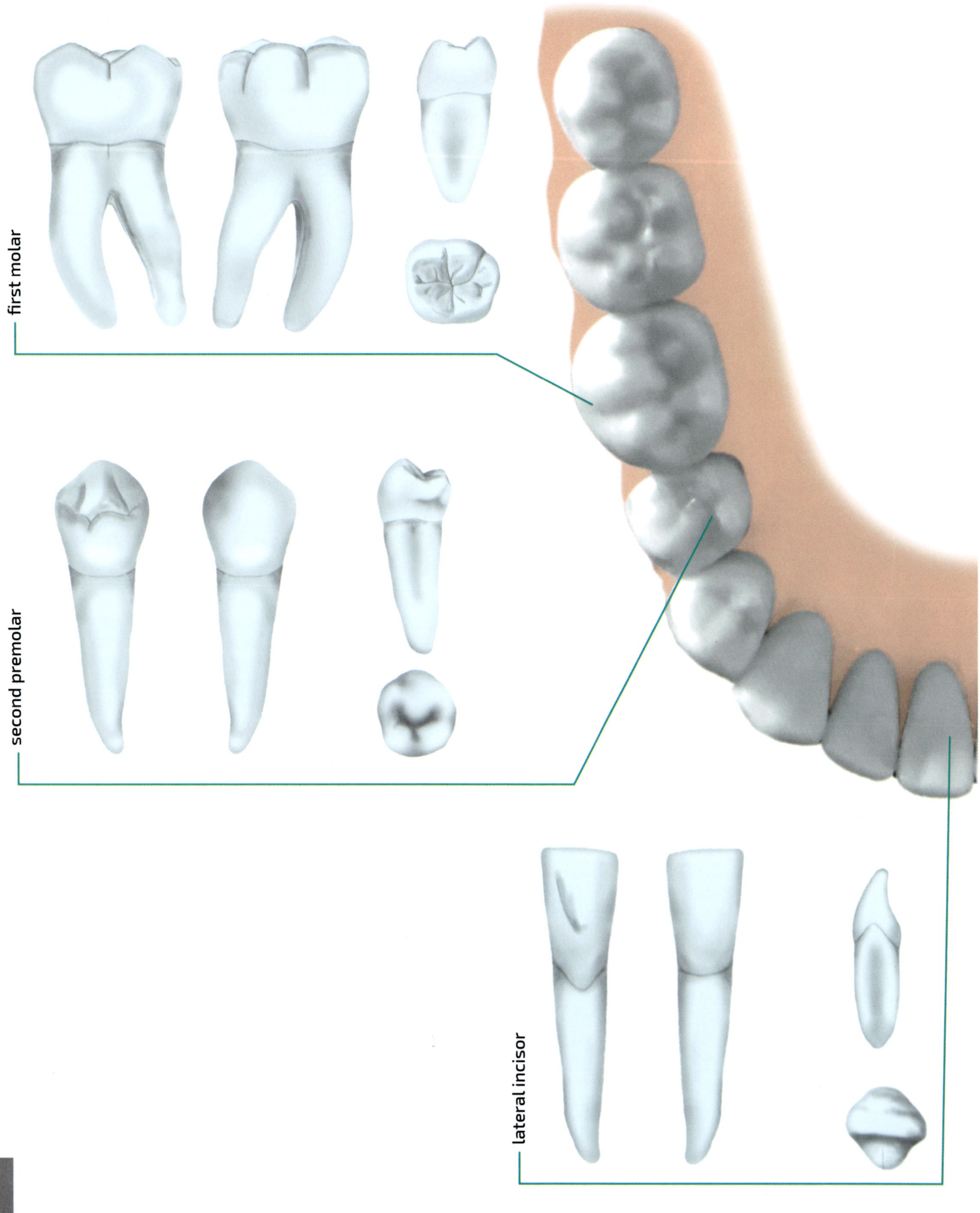
first molar
second premolar
lateral incisor

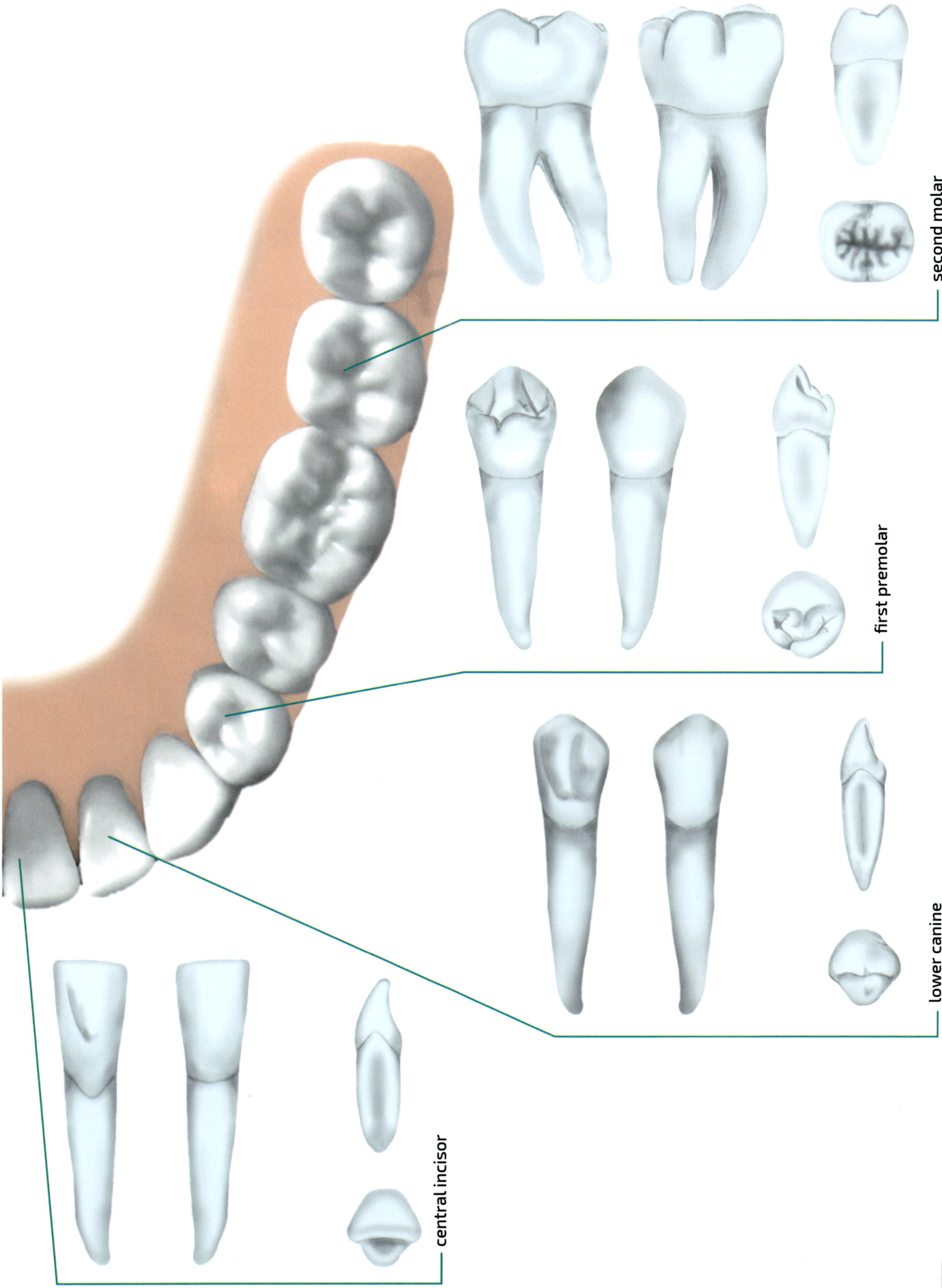
second molar
first premolar
lower canine
central incisor

ERUPTION TIMES DECIDUOUS TEETH

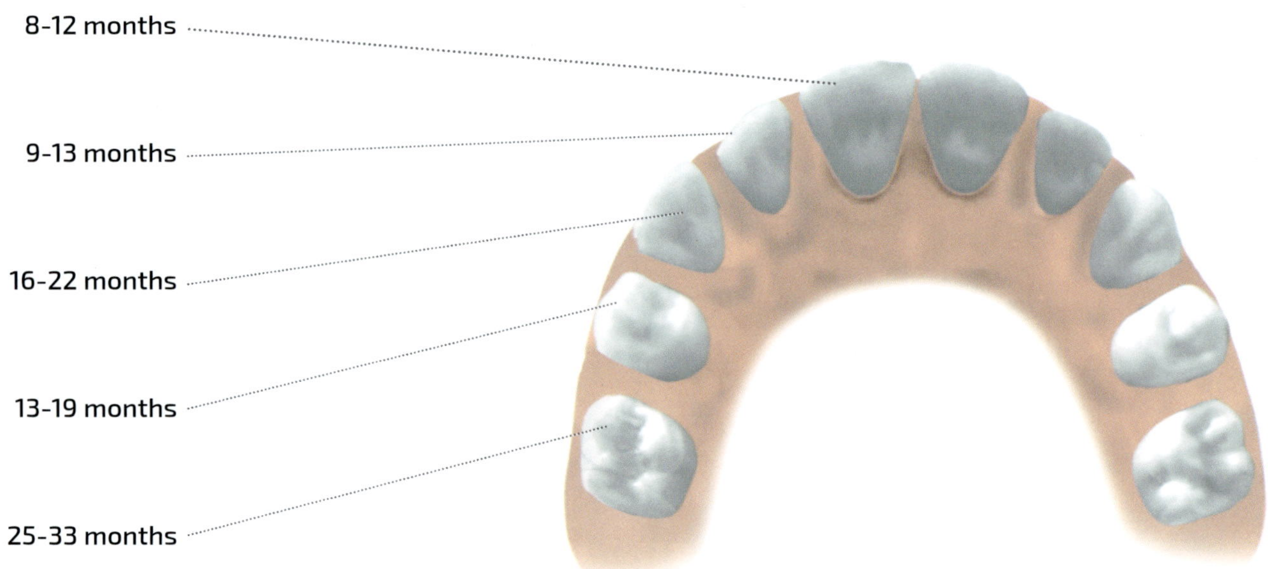

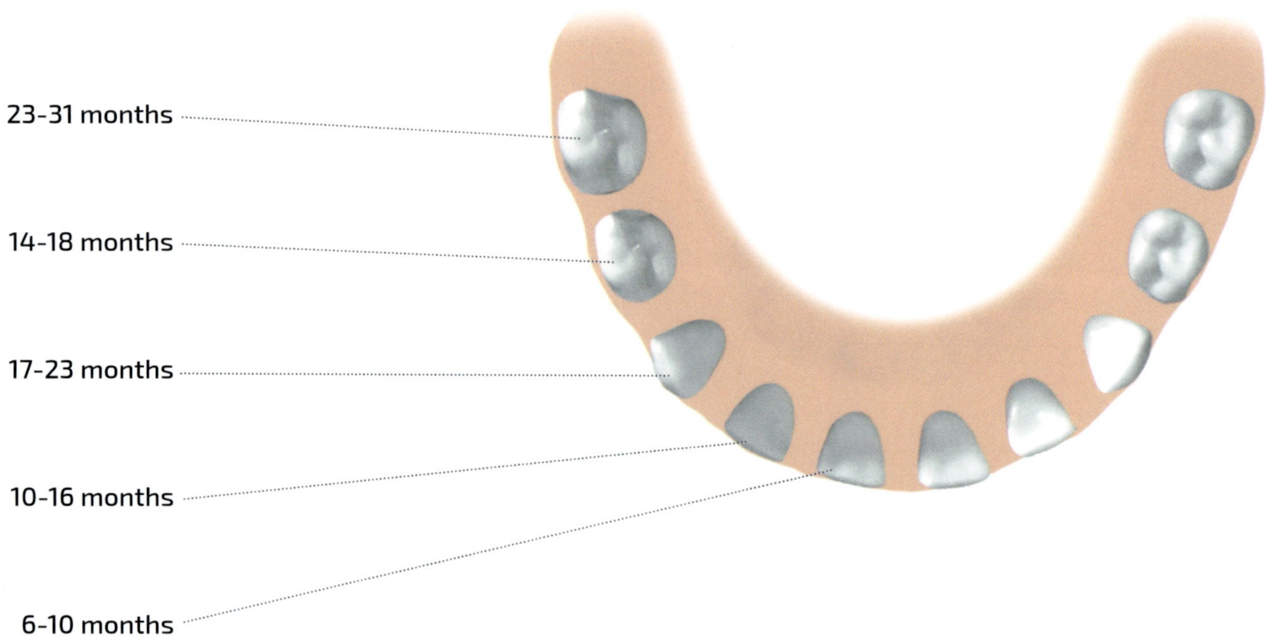

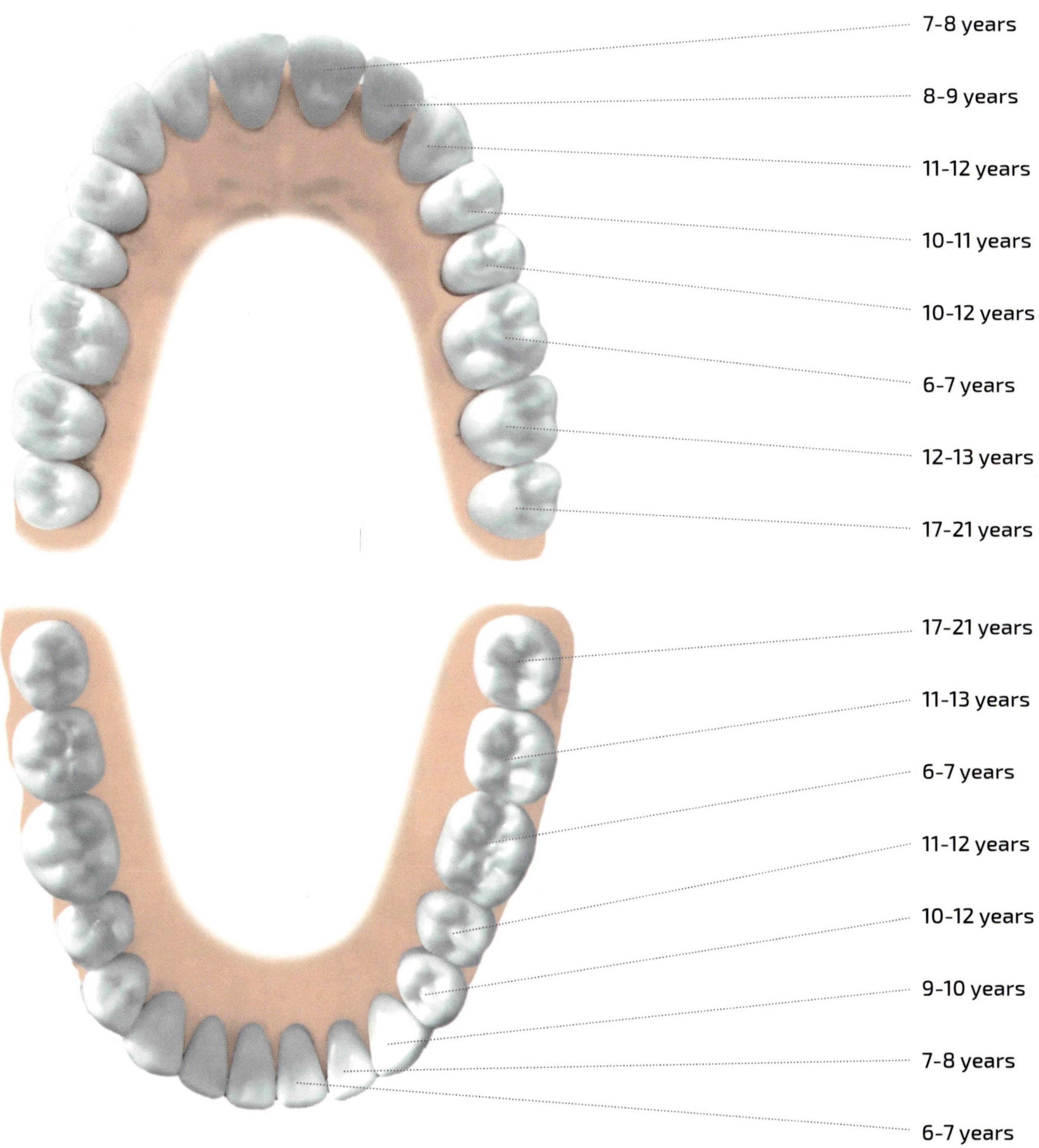
7-8 years
8-9 years
11-12 years
10-11 years
10-12 years
6-7 years
12-13 years
17-21 years
17-21 years
11-13 years
6-7 years
11-12 years
10-12 years
9-10 years
7-8 years
6-7 years

SINGLE IMPLANT AND SCREW-RETAINED OR CEMENTED CROWN

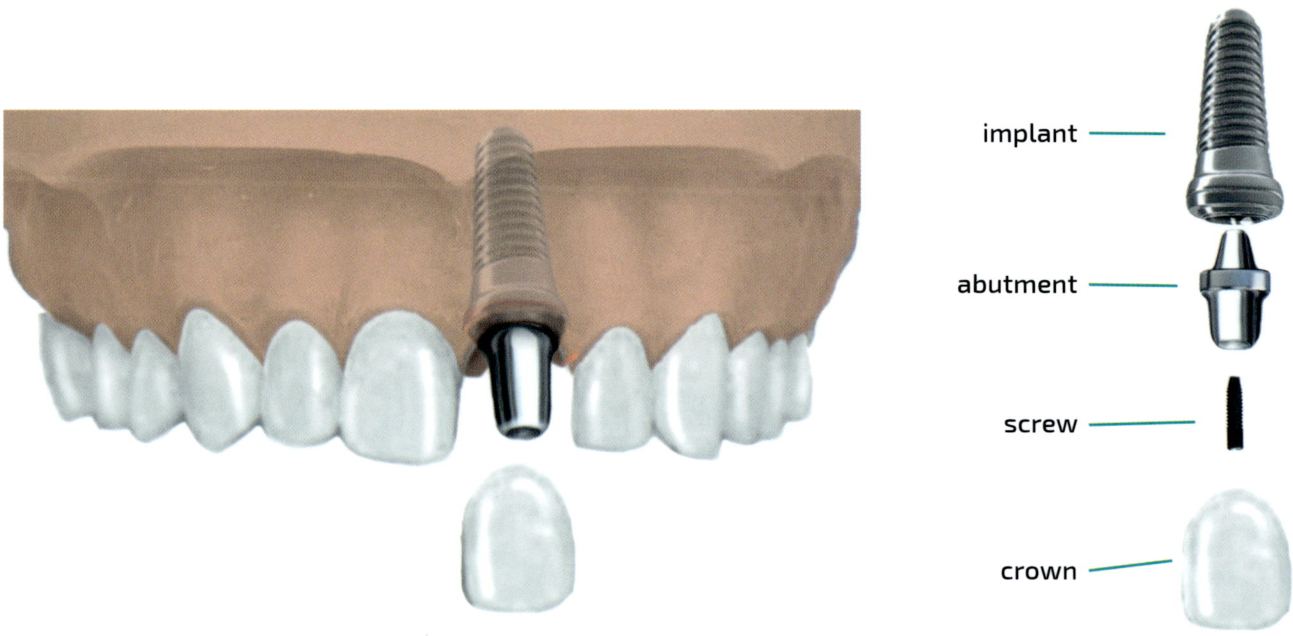

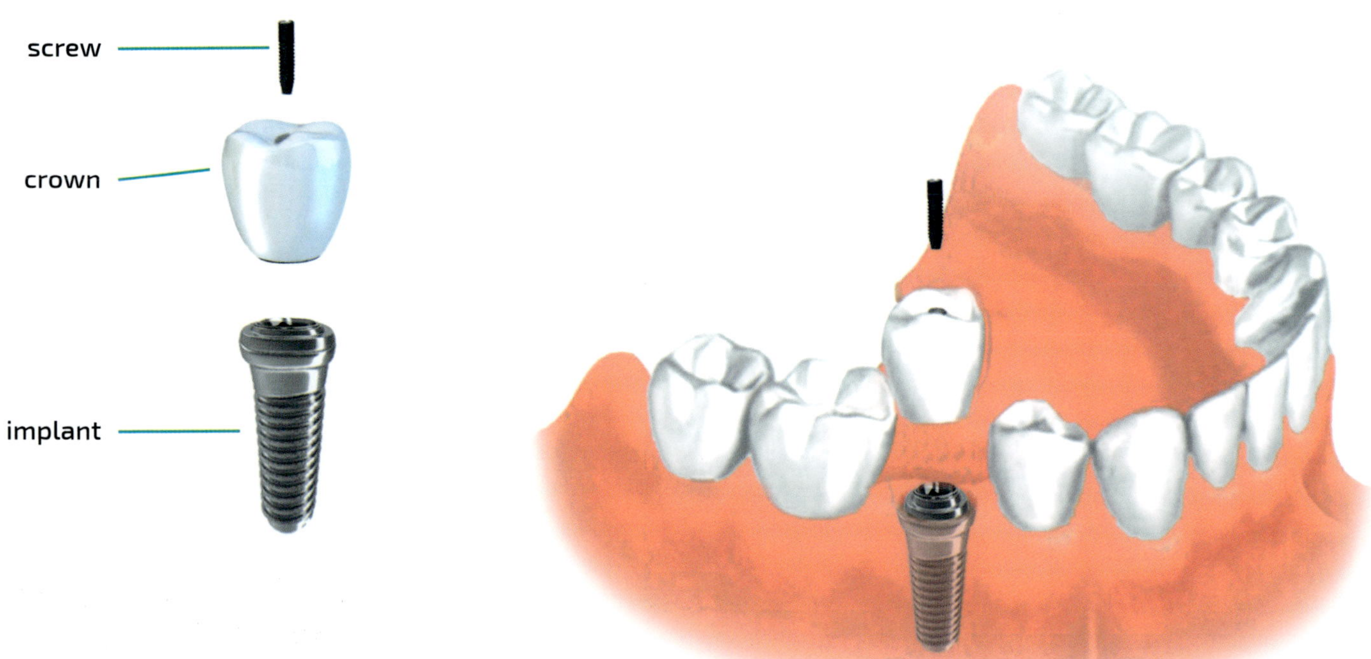

Rehabilitation of a missing tooth.
It consists of the insertion inside of the alveolar bone of an implant to which a prosthetic crown is connected by screw-retained or cemented techniques.

3-ELEMENT BRIDGE SCREWED/CEMENTED ON TWO IMPLANTS

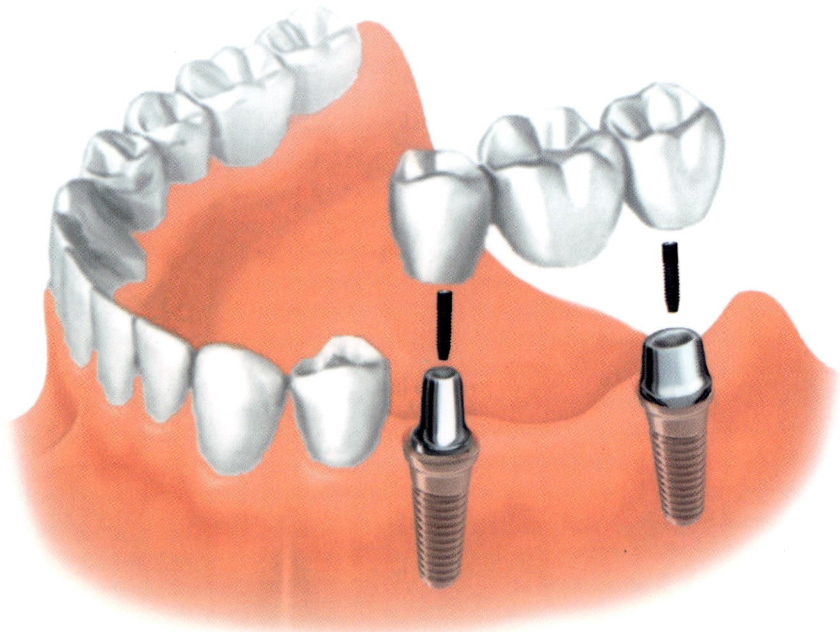

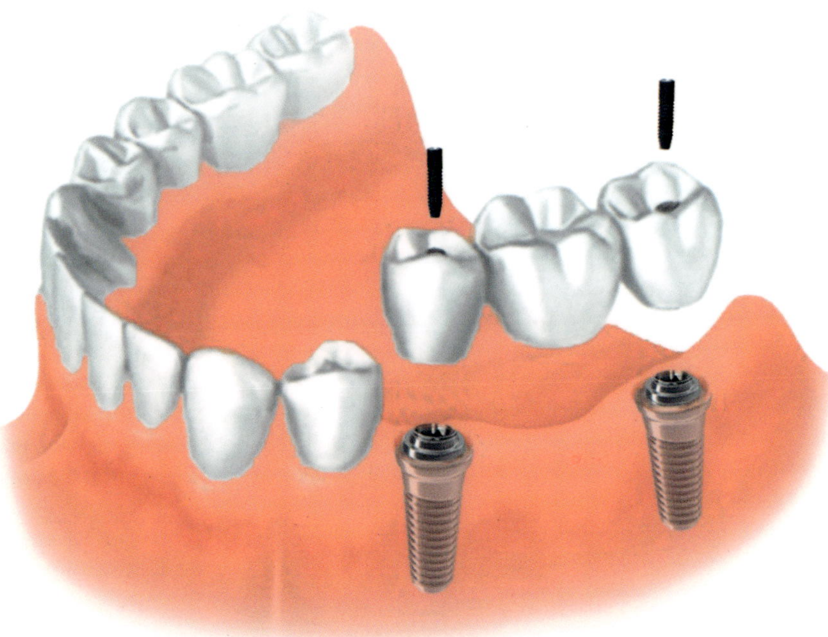

Rehabilitation with three prosthetic elements cemented (above) or screw-retained (below) on two implants.

IMPLANTOLOGY

TOTAL MOBILE PROSTHESIS ON TWO IMPLANTS

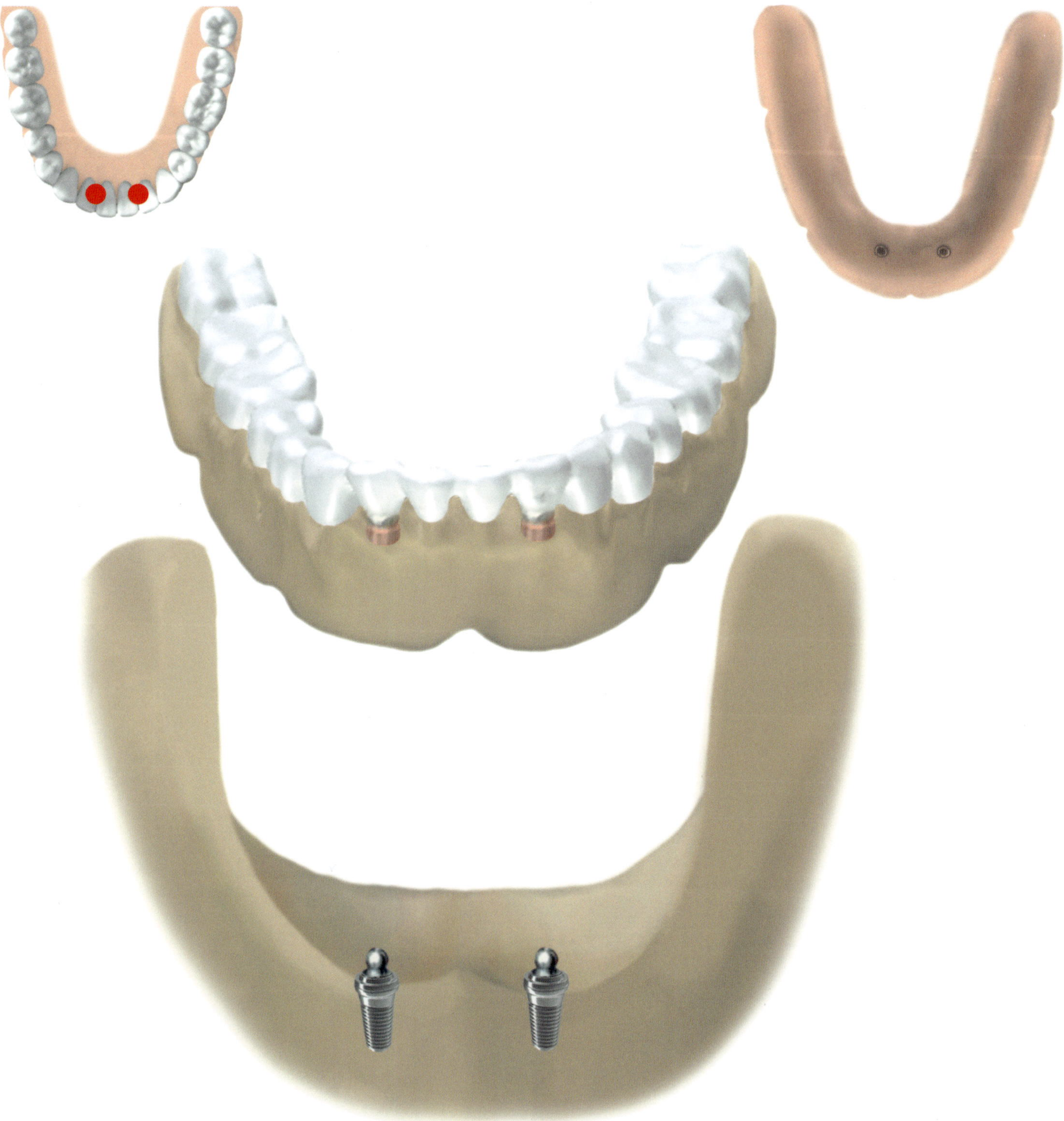

Lower total mobile prosthesis, stabilized by two implants equipped with ball attachment.

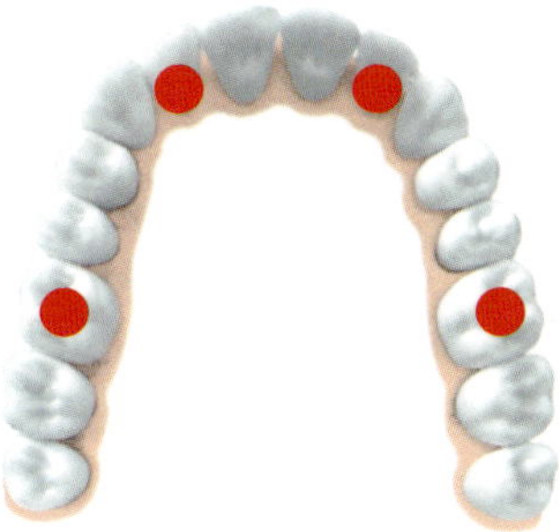

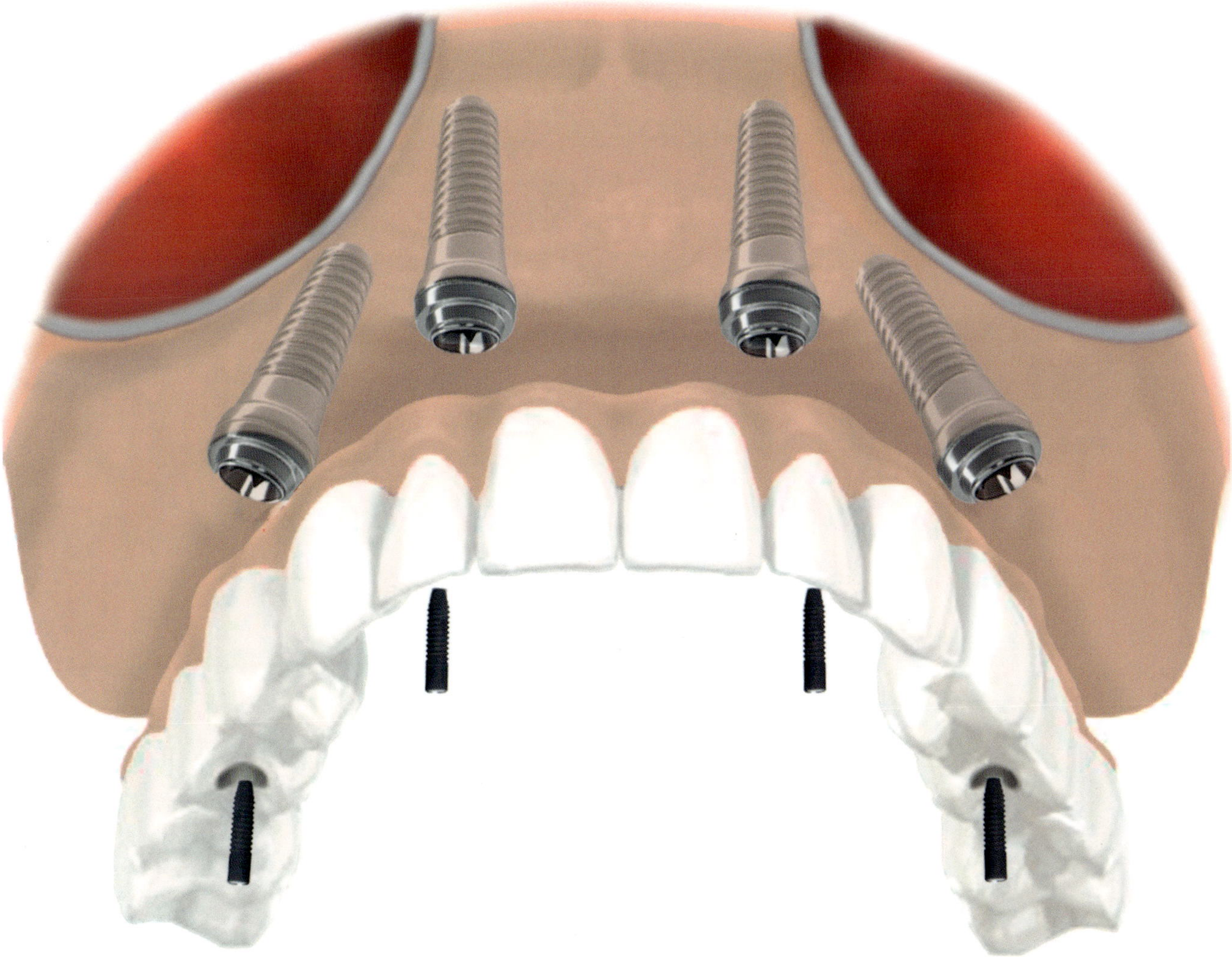

Toronto bridge-type prosthetic rehabilitation
of the entire upper arch supported by four implants.

UPPER ALL-ON-4 WITH BAR AND OVERDENTURE

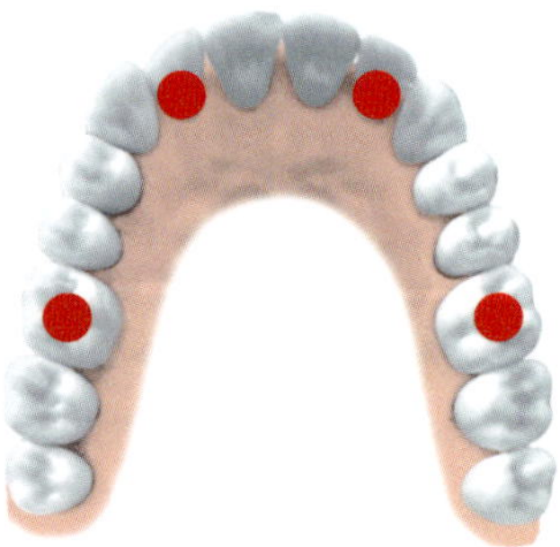

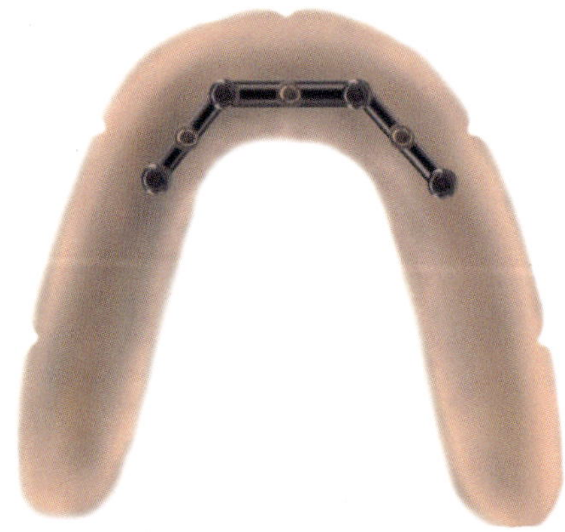

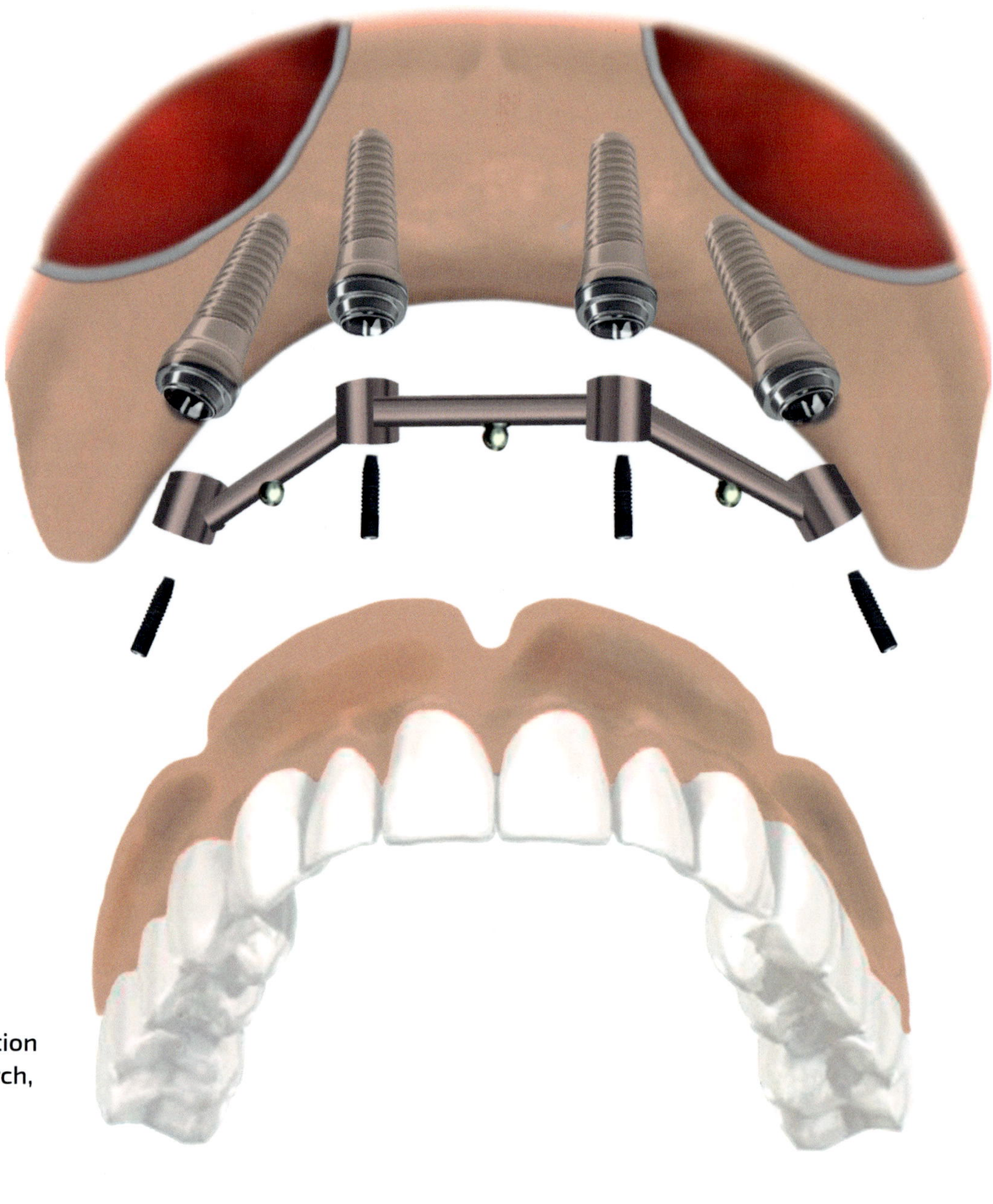

Overdenture-type prosthetic rehabilitation of the entire upper arch, with a bar supported by four implants.

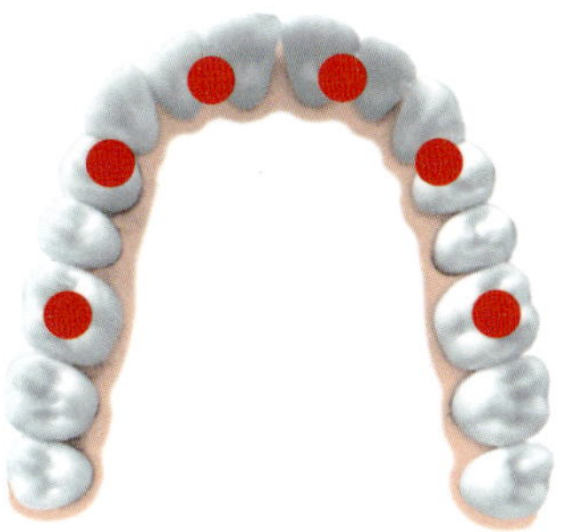

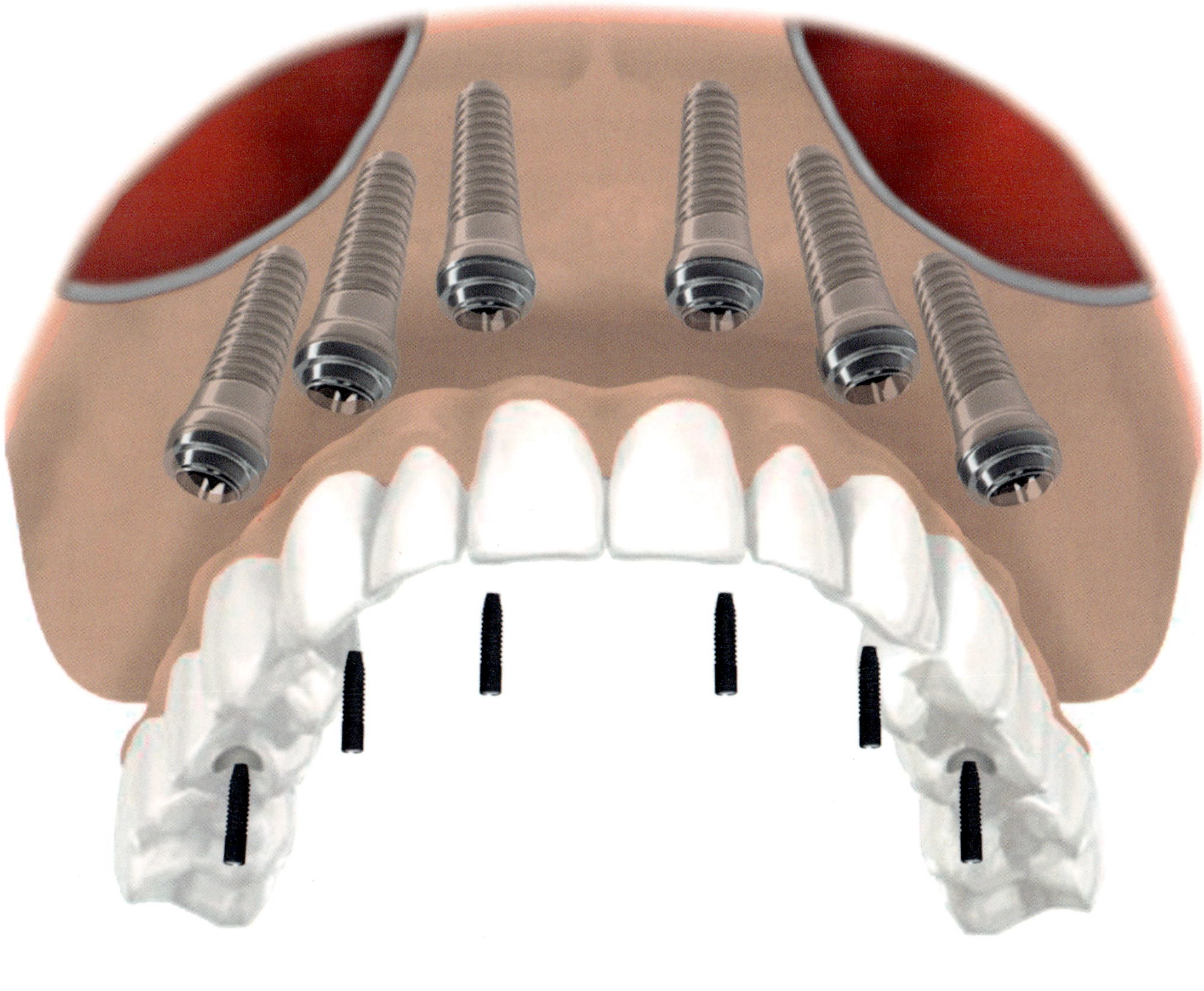

Toronto bridge-type prosthetic rehabilitation of the entire upper arch supported by six implants.

UPPER ALL-ON-6 WITH BAR AND OVERDENTURE

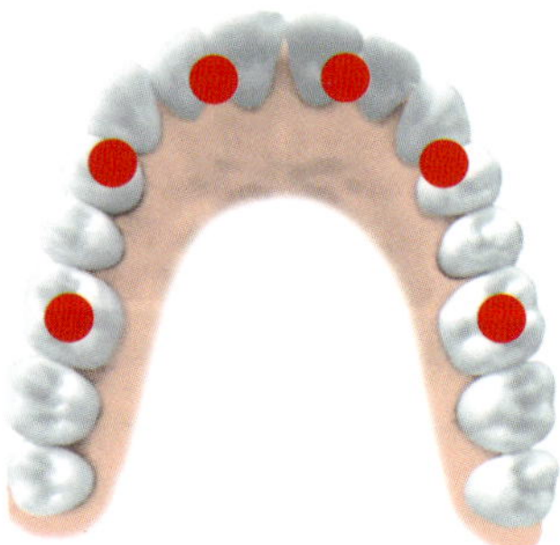

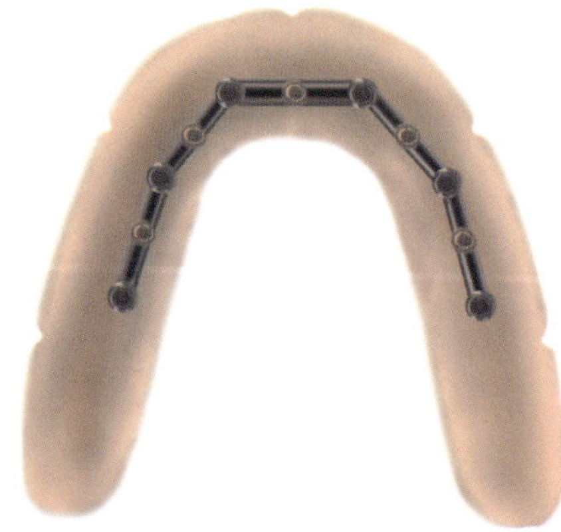

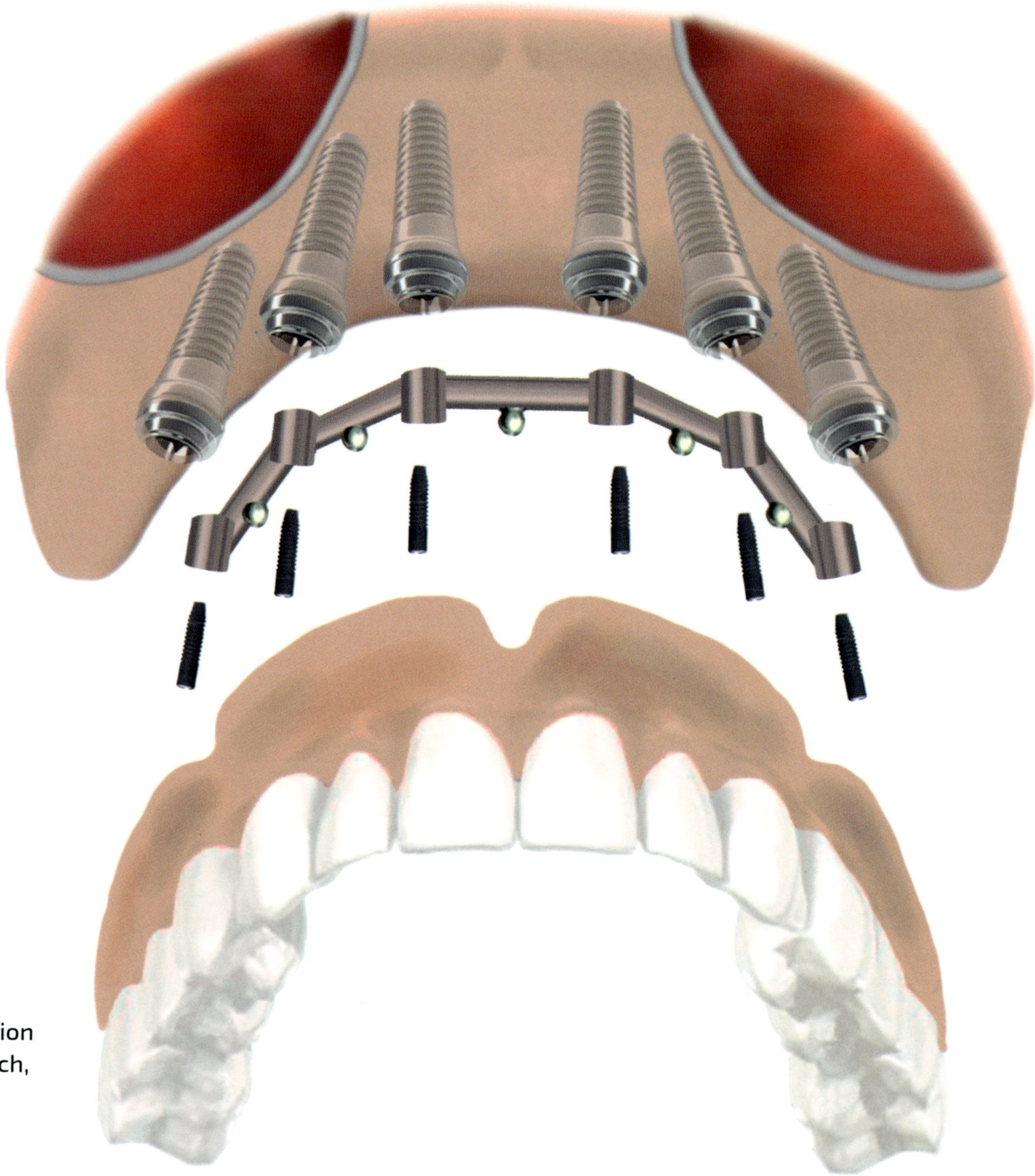

Overdenture-type prosthetic rehabilitation of the entire upper arch, with a bar supported by six implants.

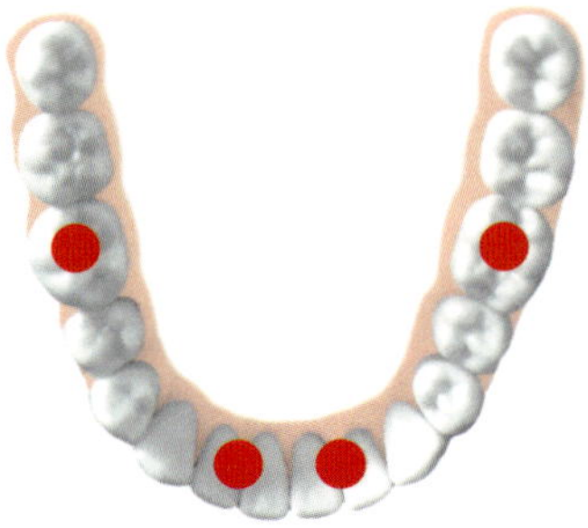

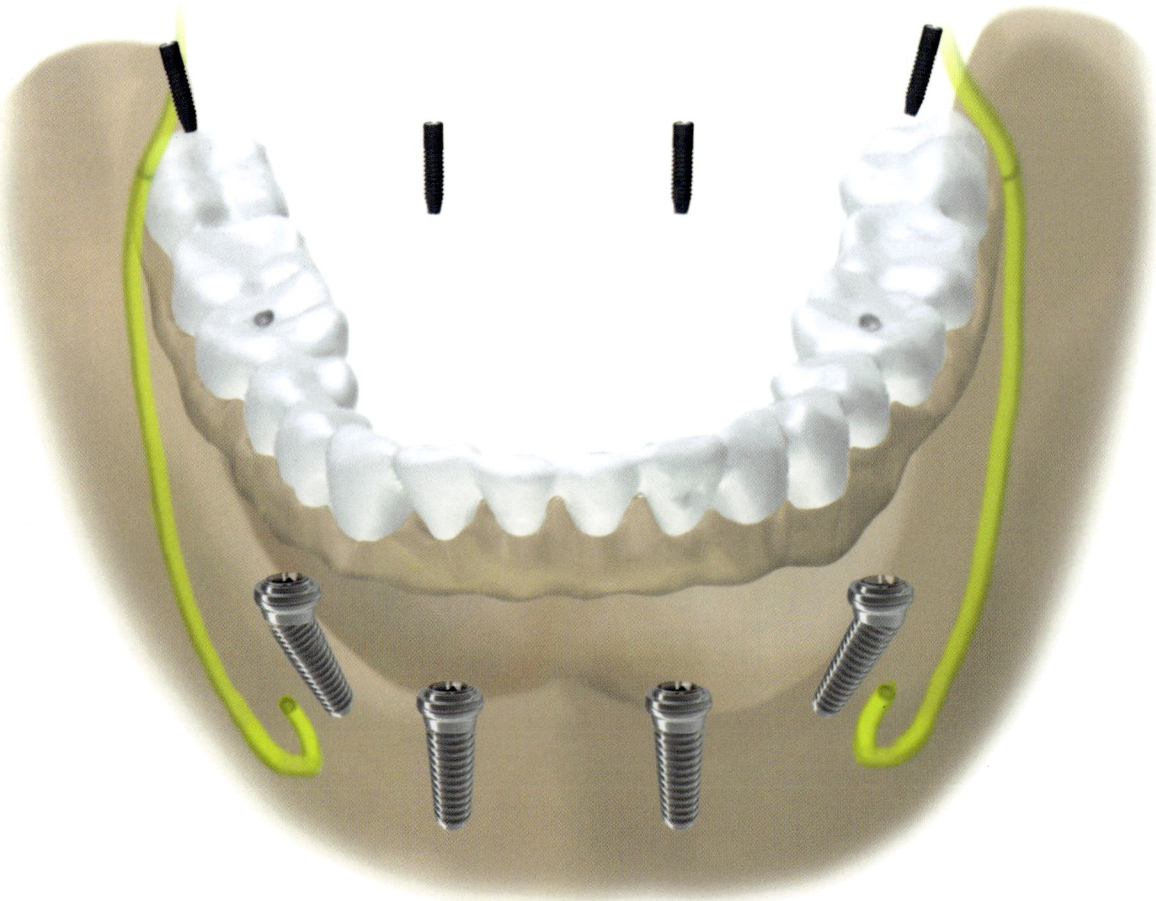

Toronto bridge-type prosthetic rehabilitation
of the entire lower arch supported by four implants.

LOWER ALL-ON-4 WITH BAR AND OVERDENTURE

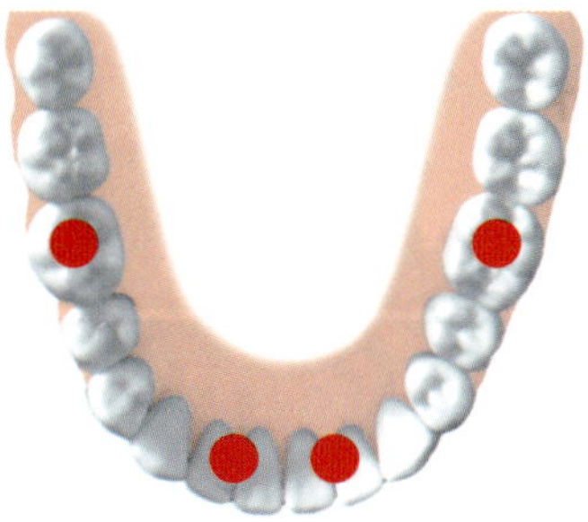

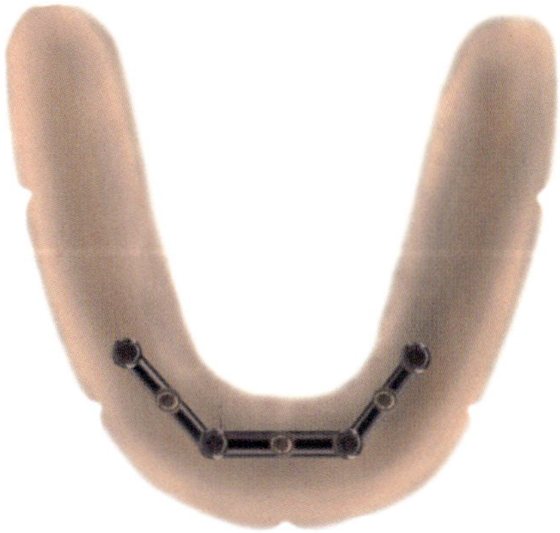

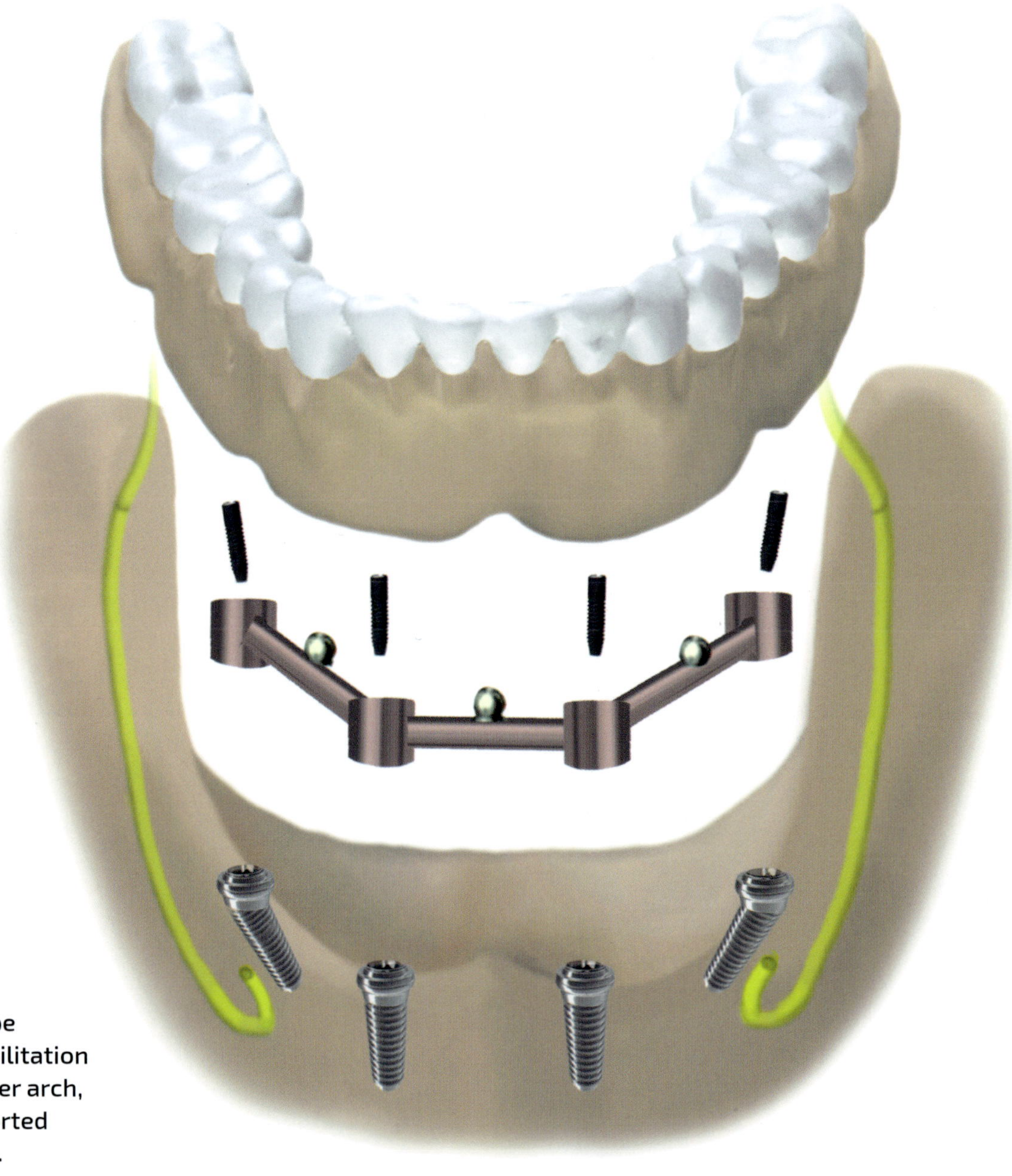

Overdenture-type prosthetic rehabilitation of the entire lower arch, with a bar supported by four implants.

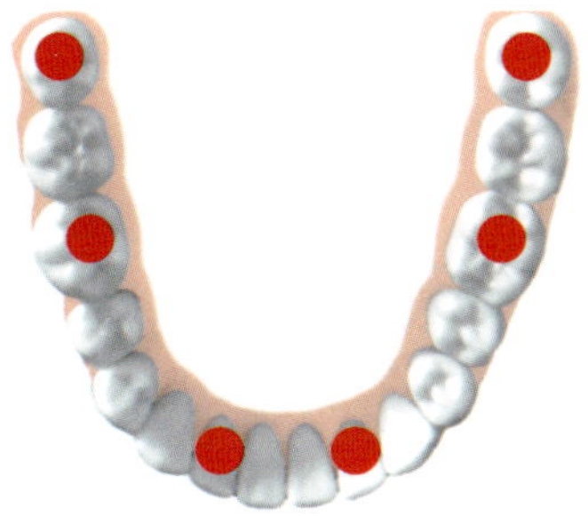

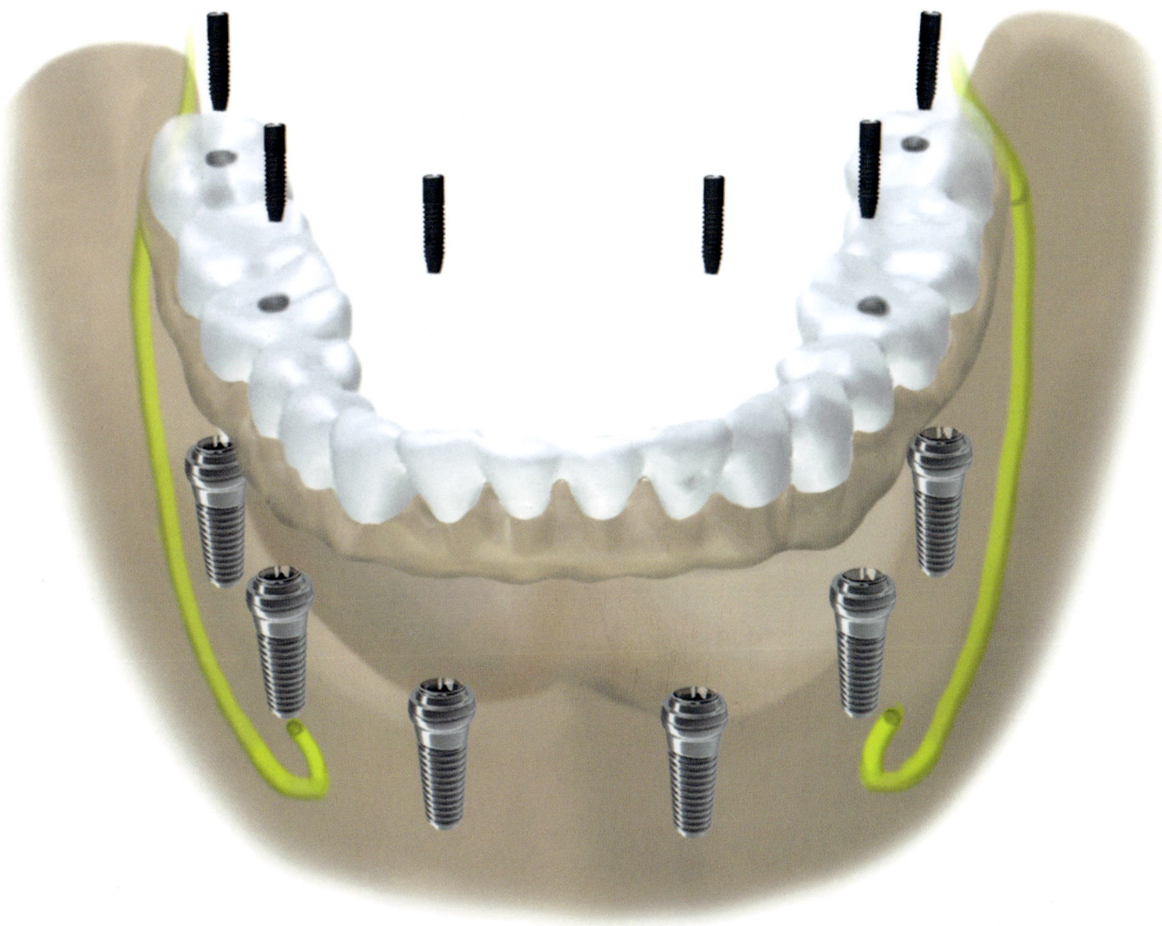

Toronto bridge-type prosthetic rehabilitation
of the entire lower arch supported by six implants.

LOWER ALL-ON-6 WITH BAR AND OVERDENTURE

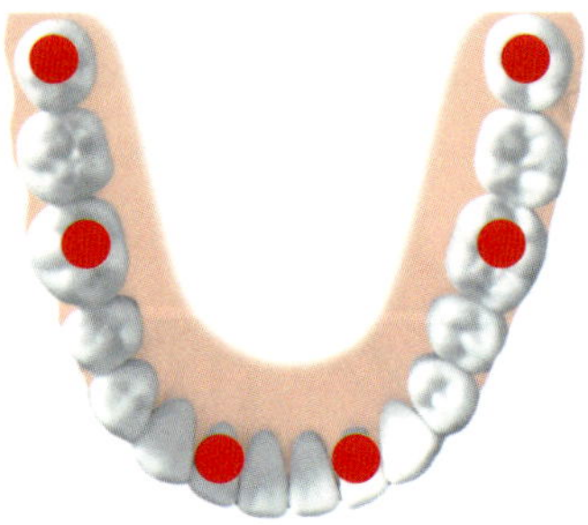

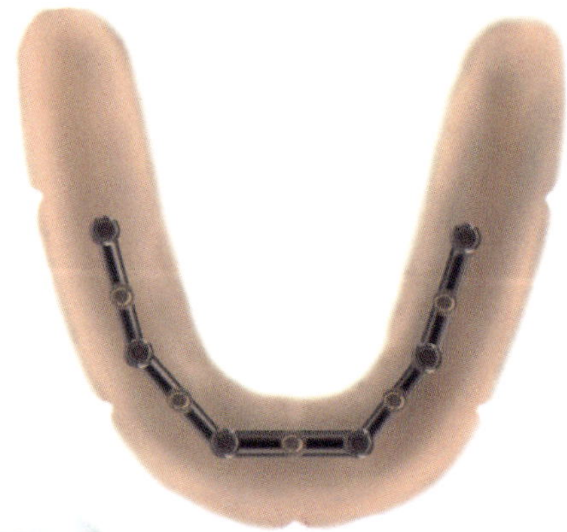

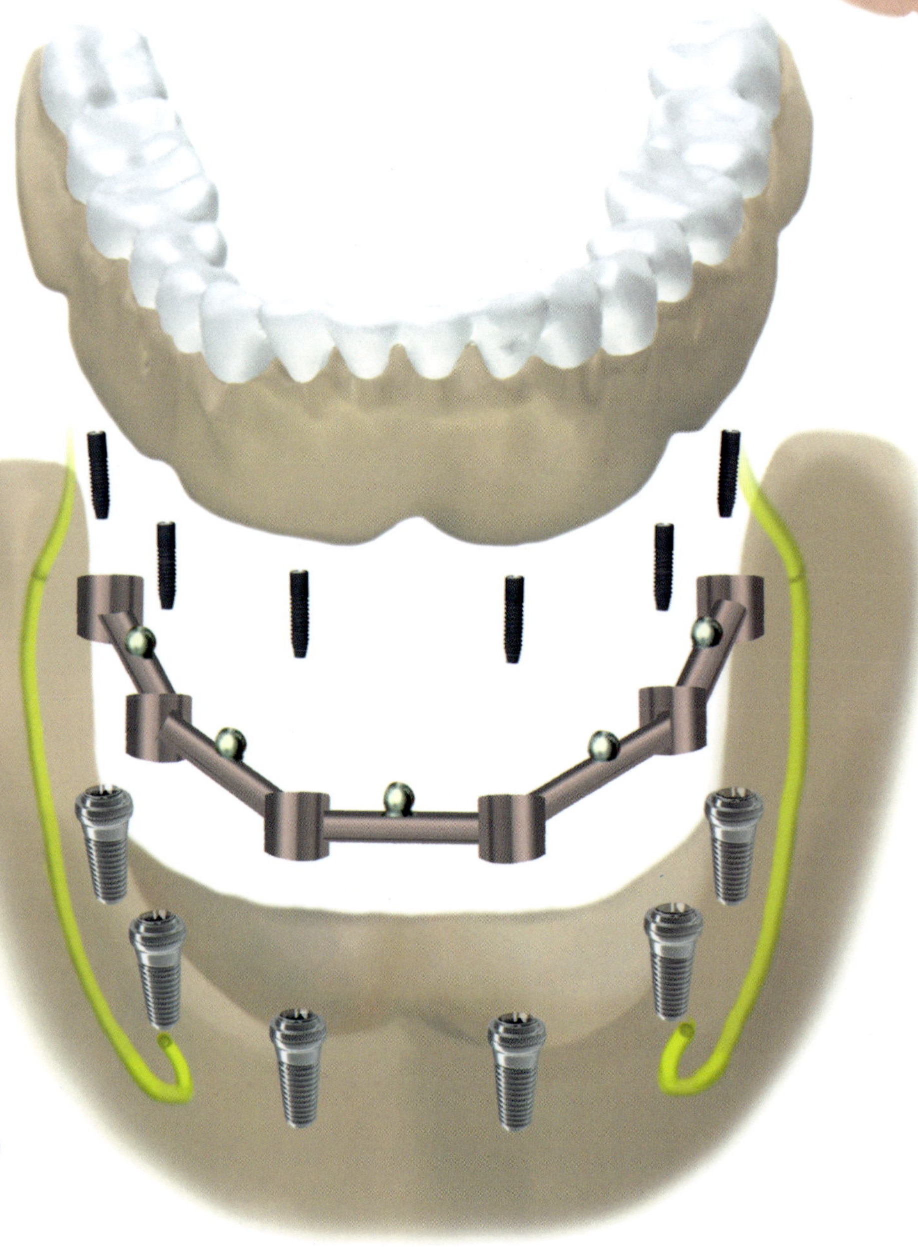

Overdenture-type prosthetic rehabilitation of the entire lower arch, with a bar supported by six implants.

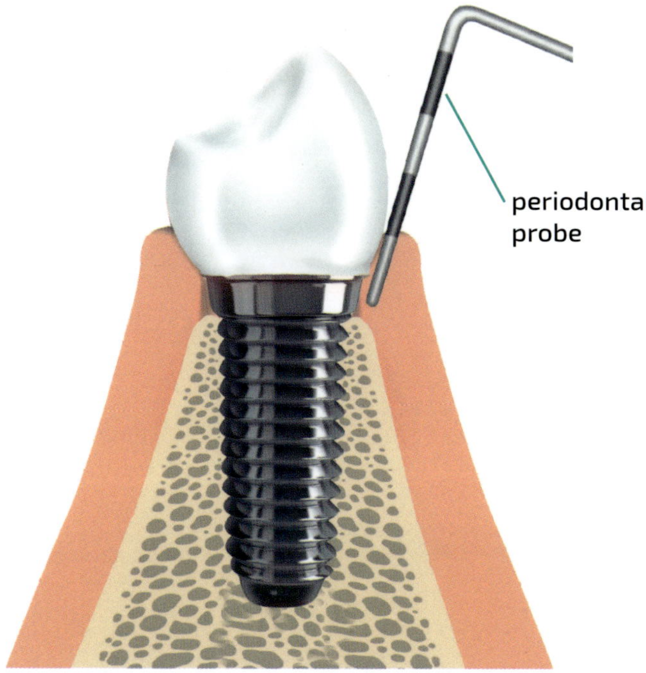

peri-implant health

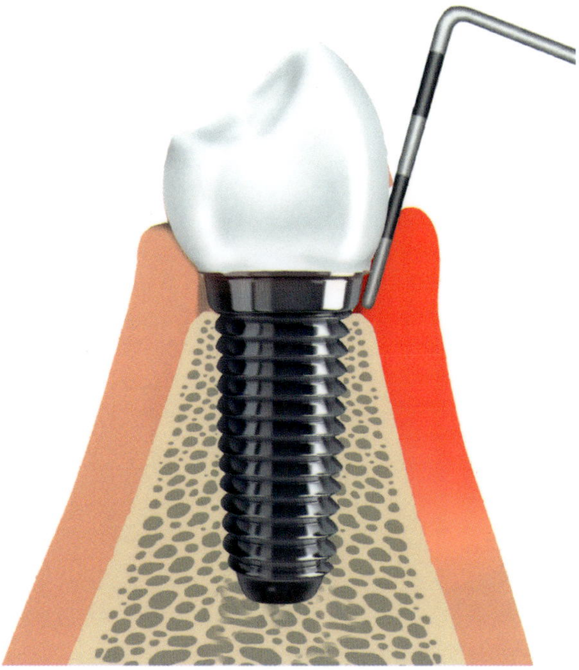

peri-implant mucositis

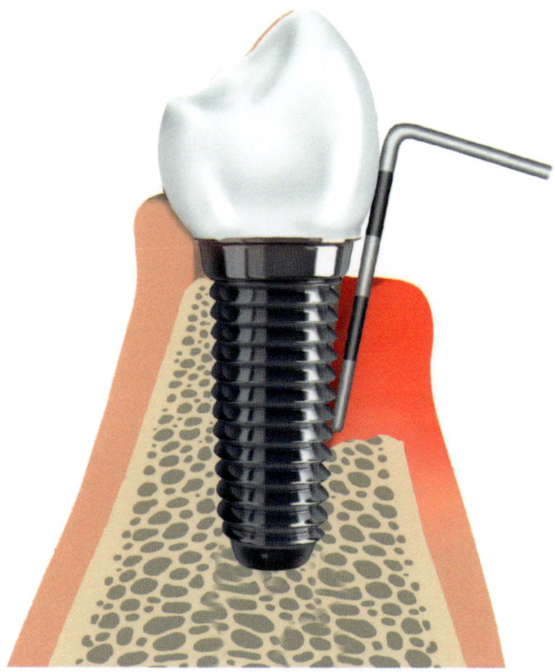

peri-implantitis

Sequence of clinical pictures leading to the onset of peri-implant disease, which is triggered by a state of peri-implant mucositis.

MINI MAXILLARY SINUS LIFT

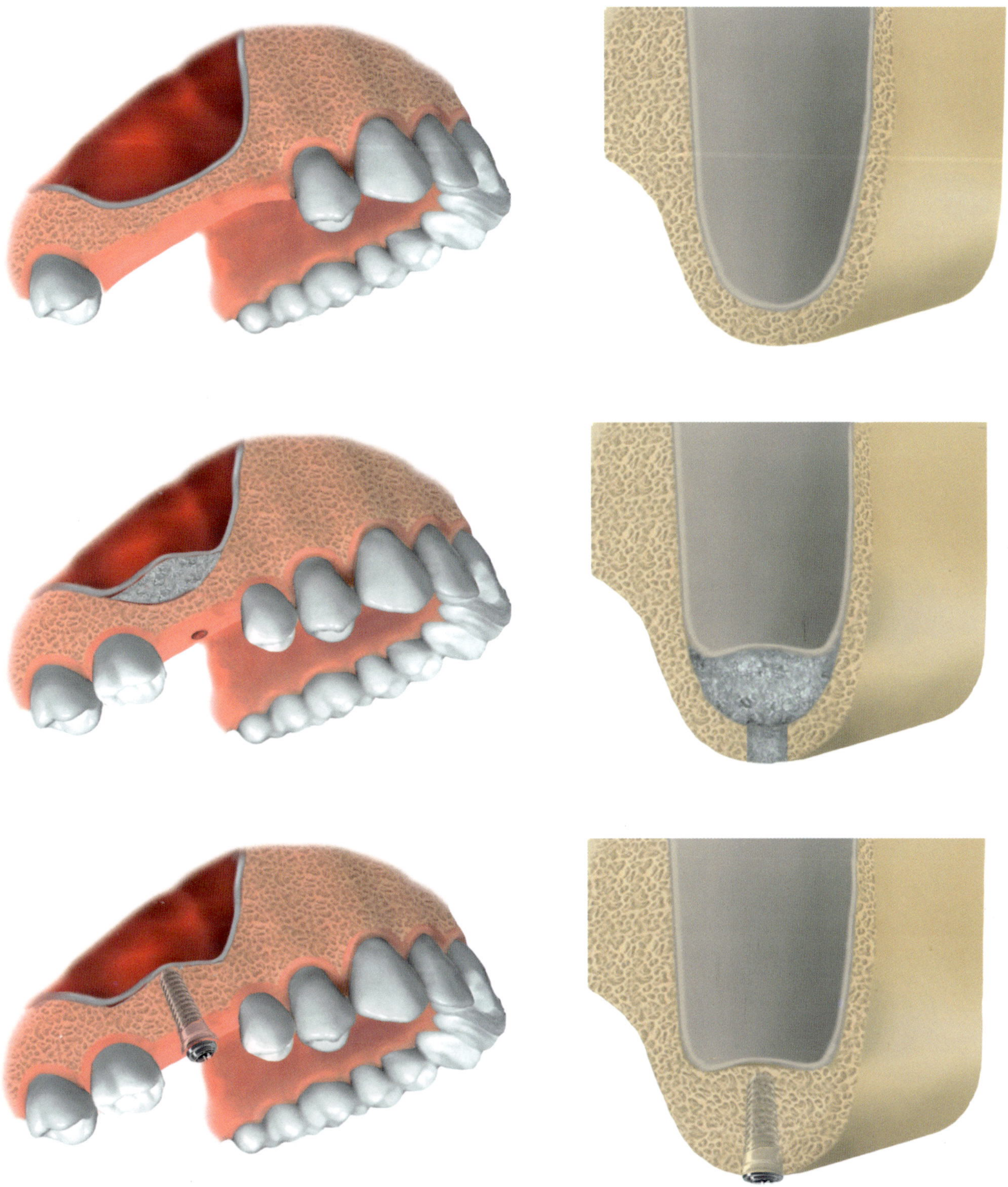

The surgery aims to increase the amount of bone tissue vertically, allowing subsequent implant insertion.

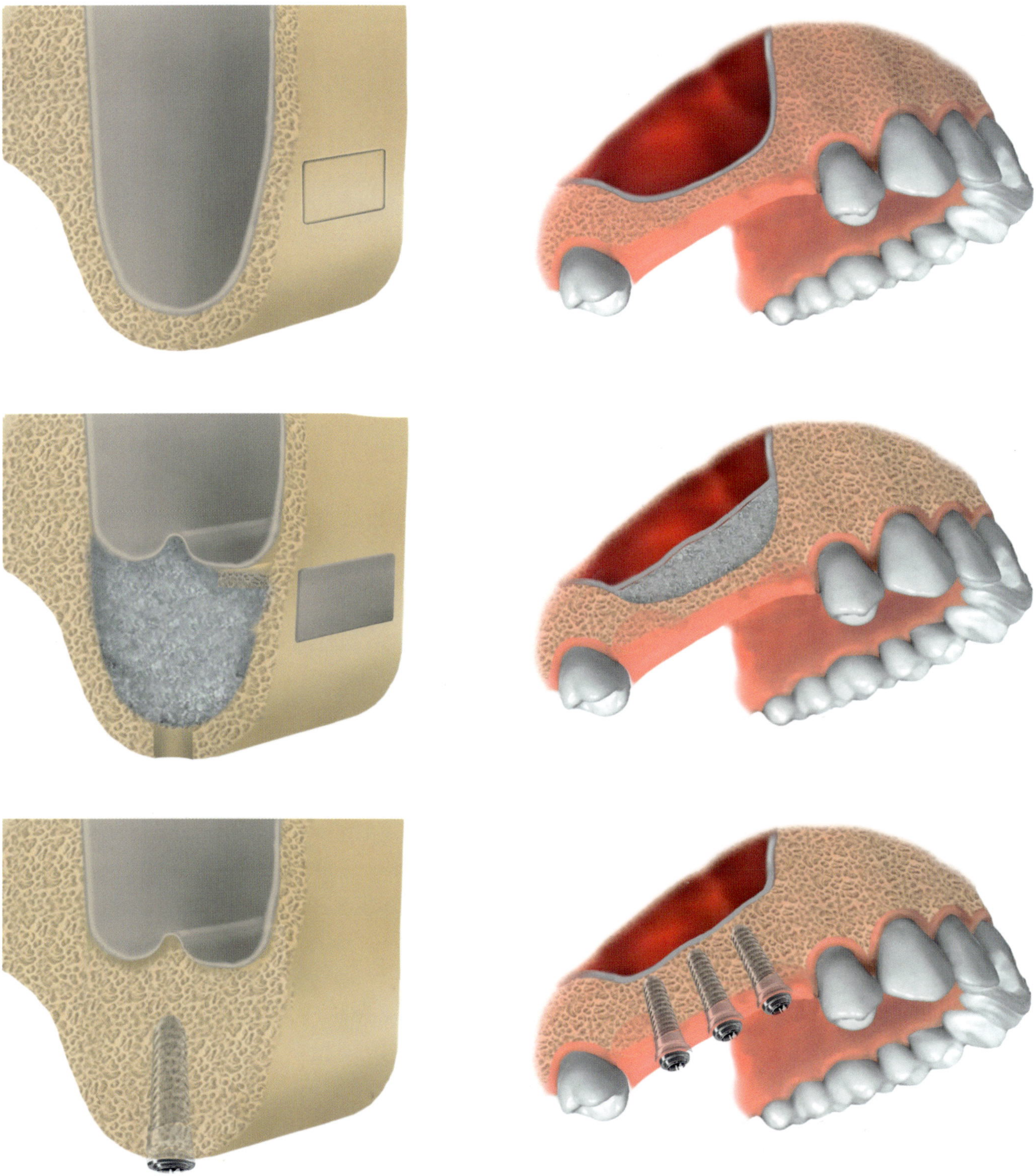

The surgery aims to increase the amount of bone tissue vertically and sometimes horizontally, allowing subsequent insertion of one or more implants.

REGENERATIVE SURGERY ON INTRAOSSEOUS DEFECT IN THE AESTHETIC AREA

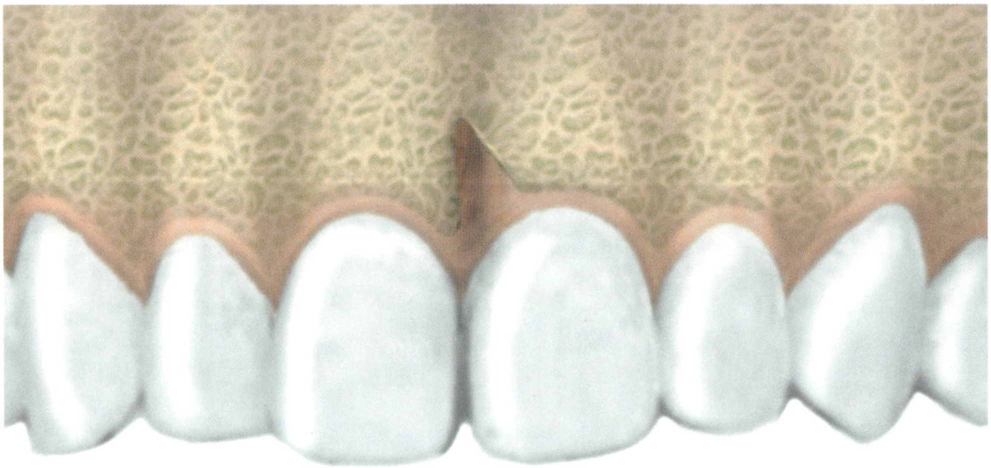

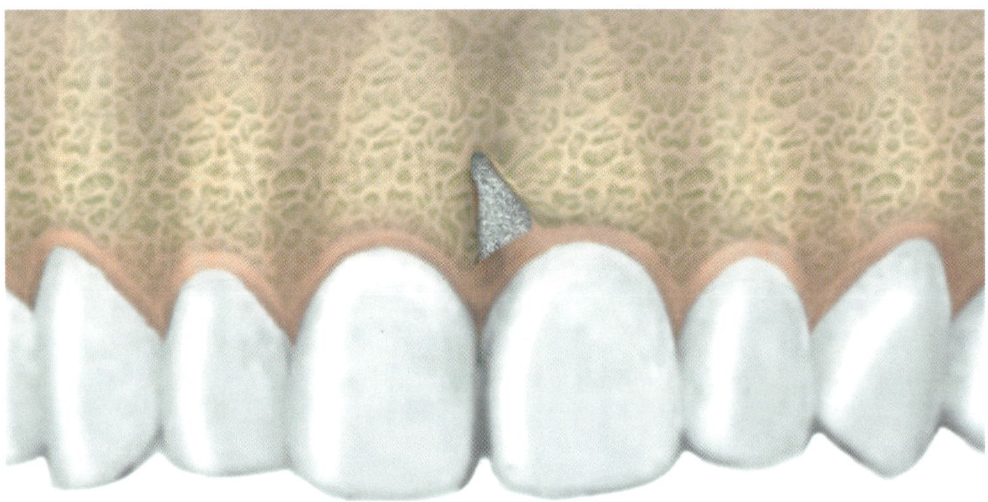

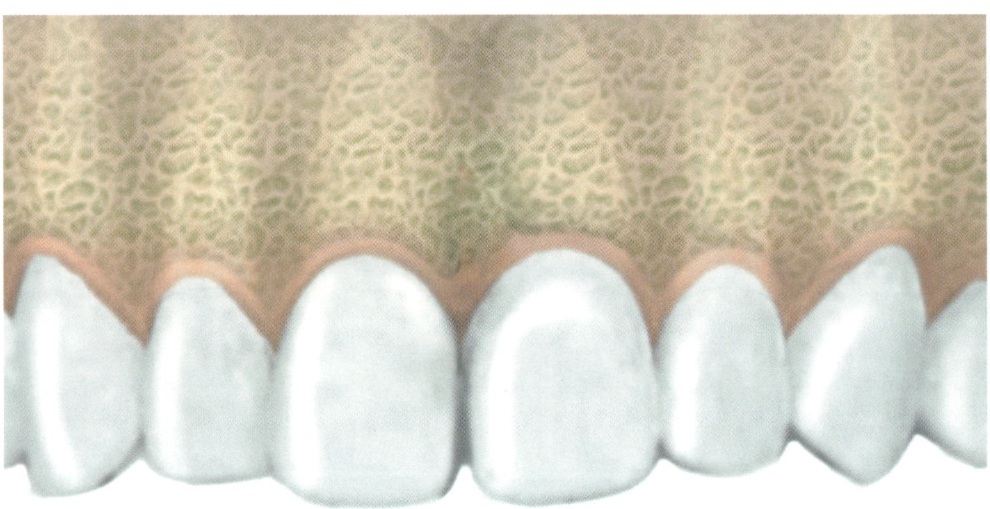

The goal of this intervention is the surgical correction of vertical resorptions in the aesthetic (anterior) area with or without the aid of bone substitutes.

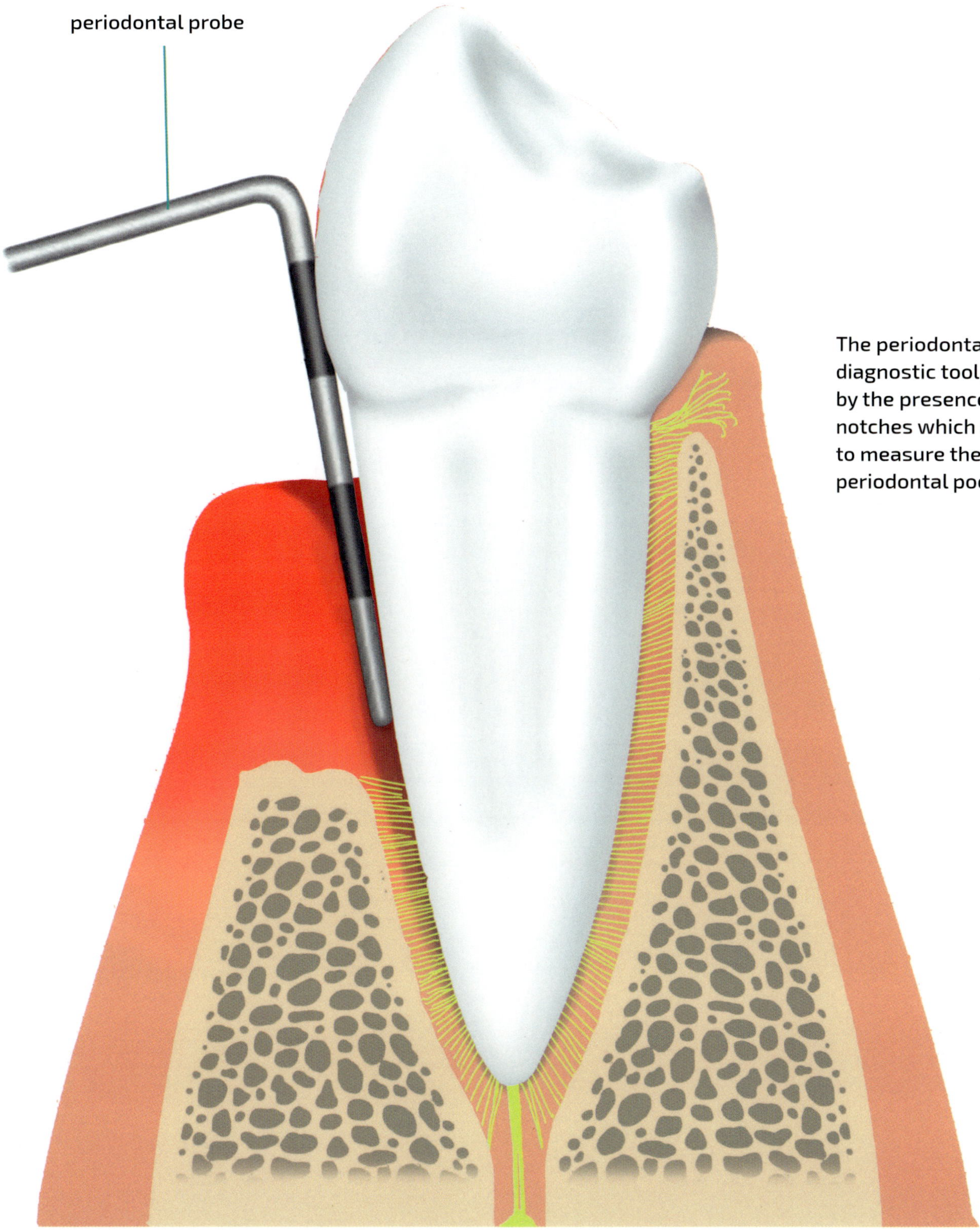

The periodontal probe is a diagnostic tool, characterized by the presence of millimeter notches which are used to measure the depth of the periodontal pockets.

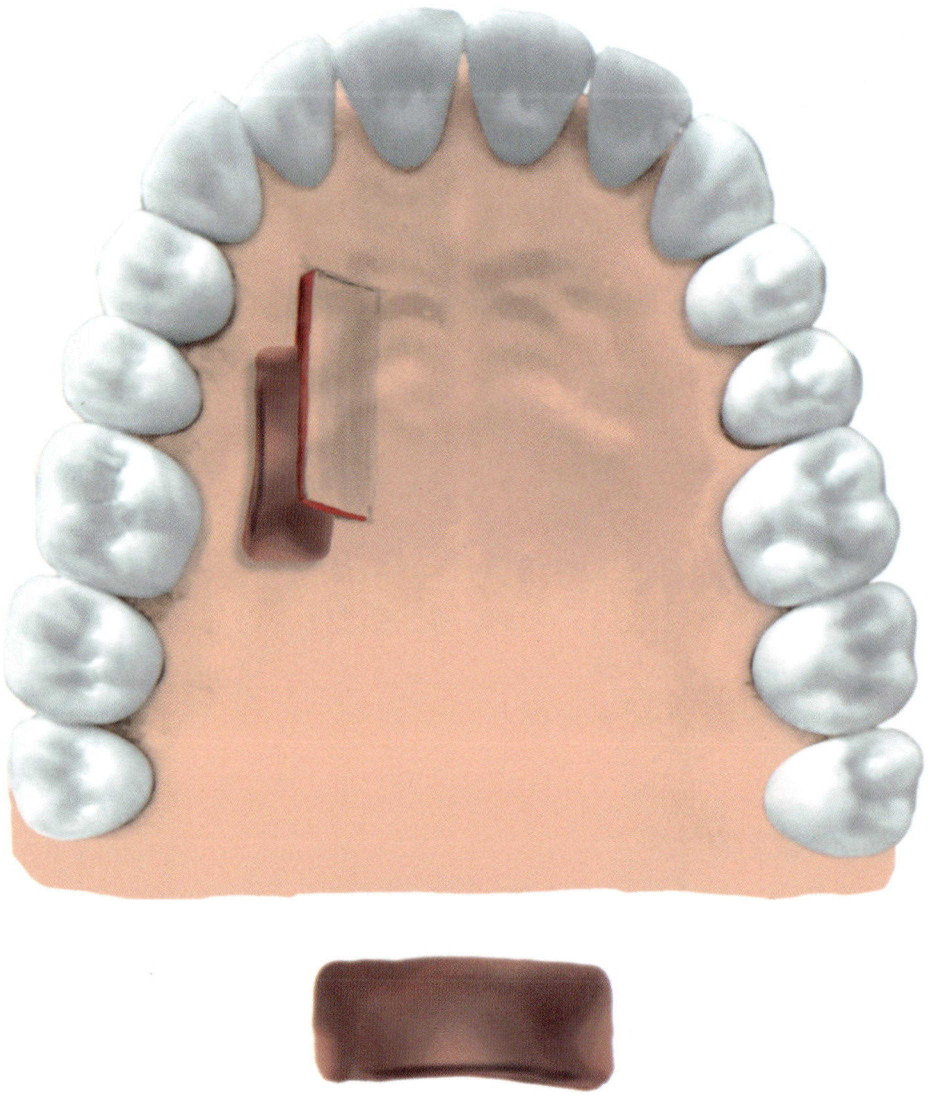

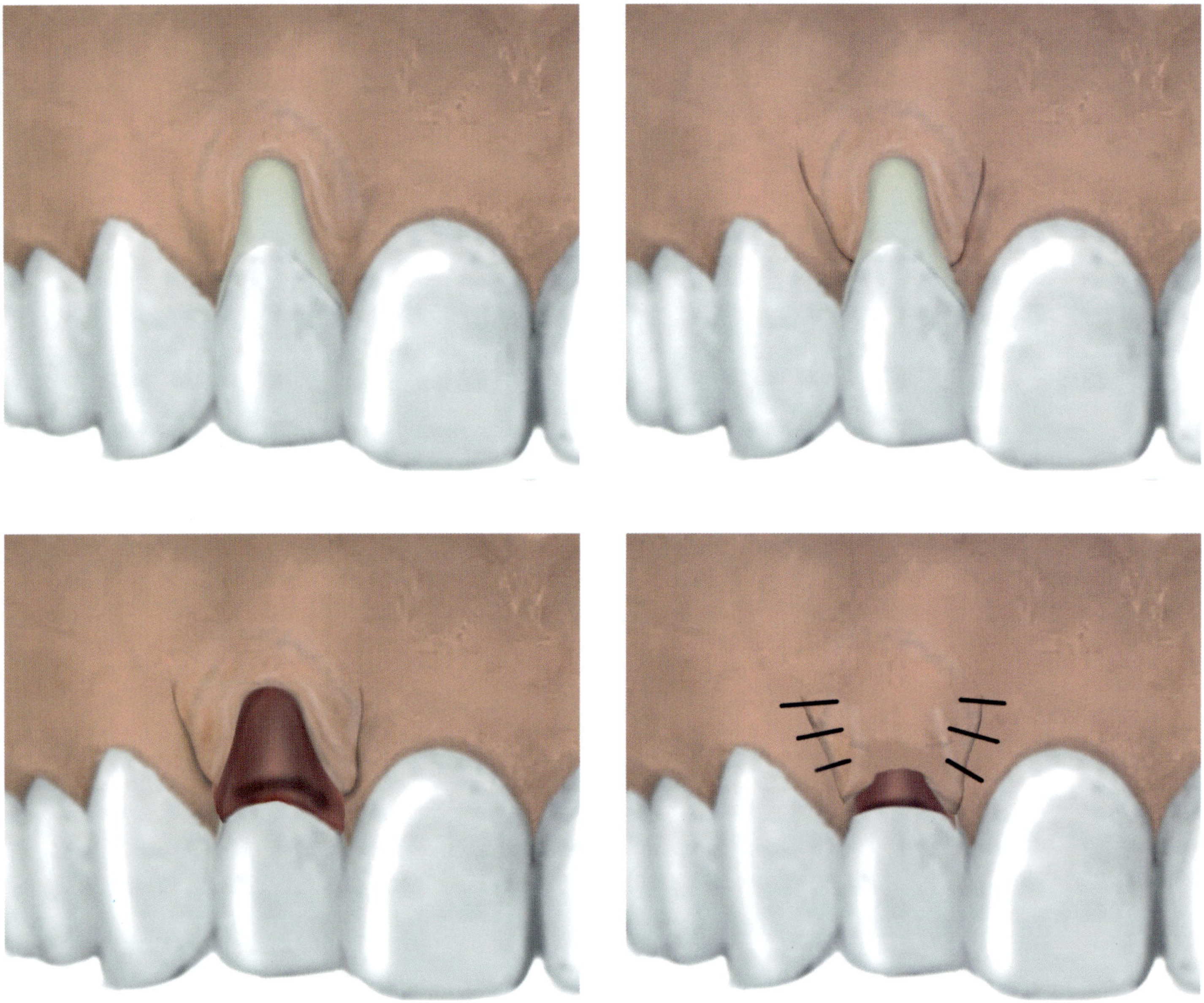

The harvested connective tissue or epithelial-connective tissue will be subsequently placed and sutured under the vestibular flap, covering the recession defect.

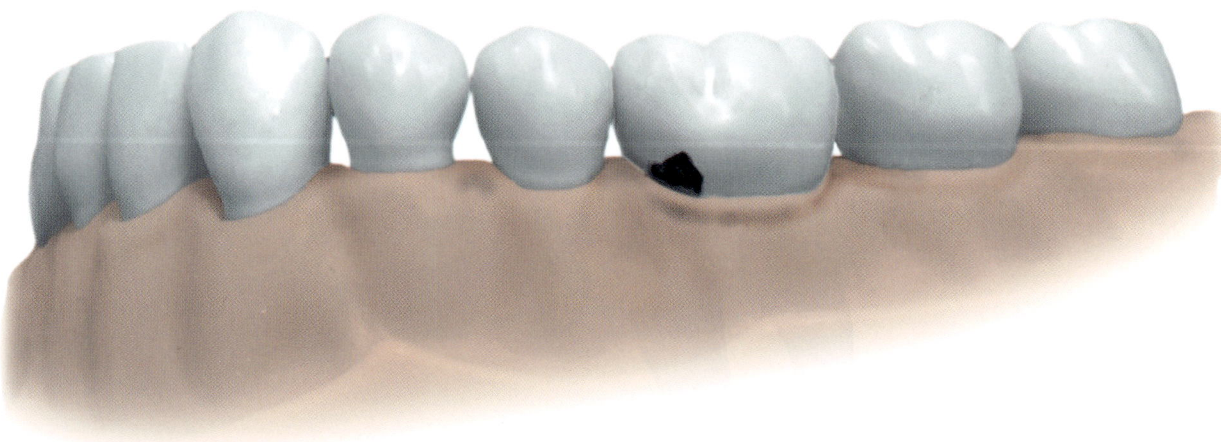

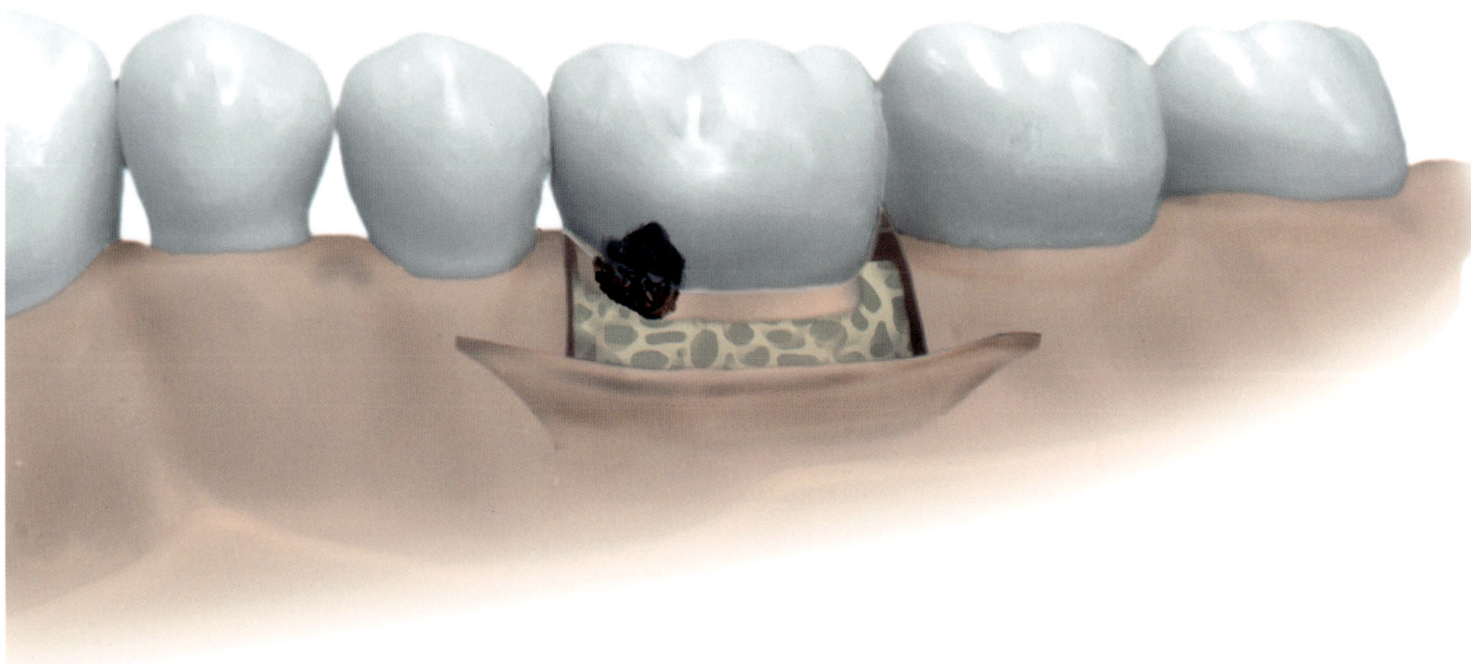

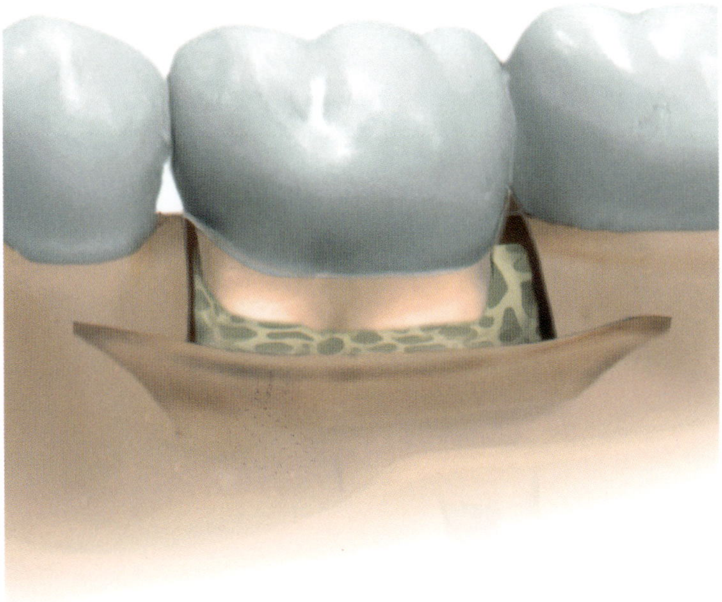
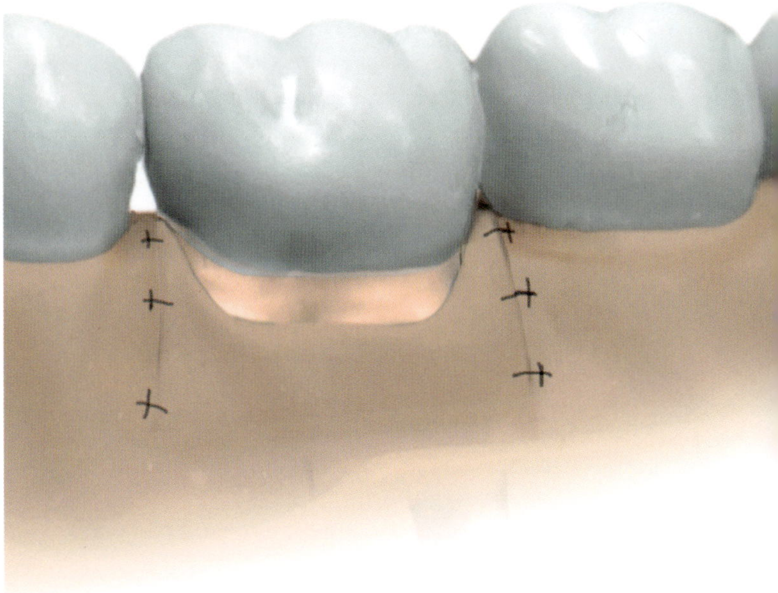
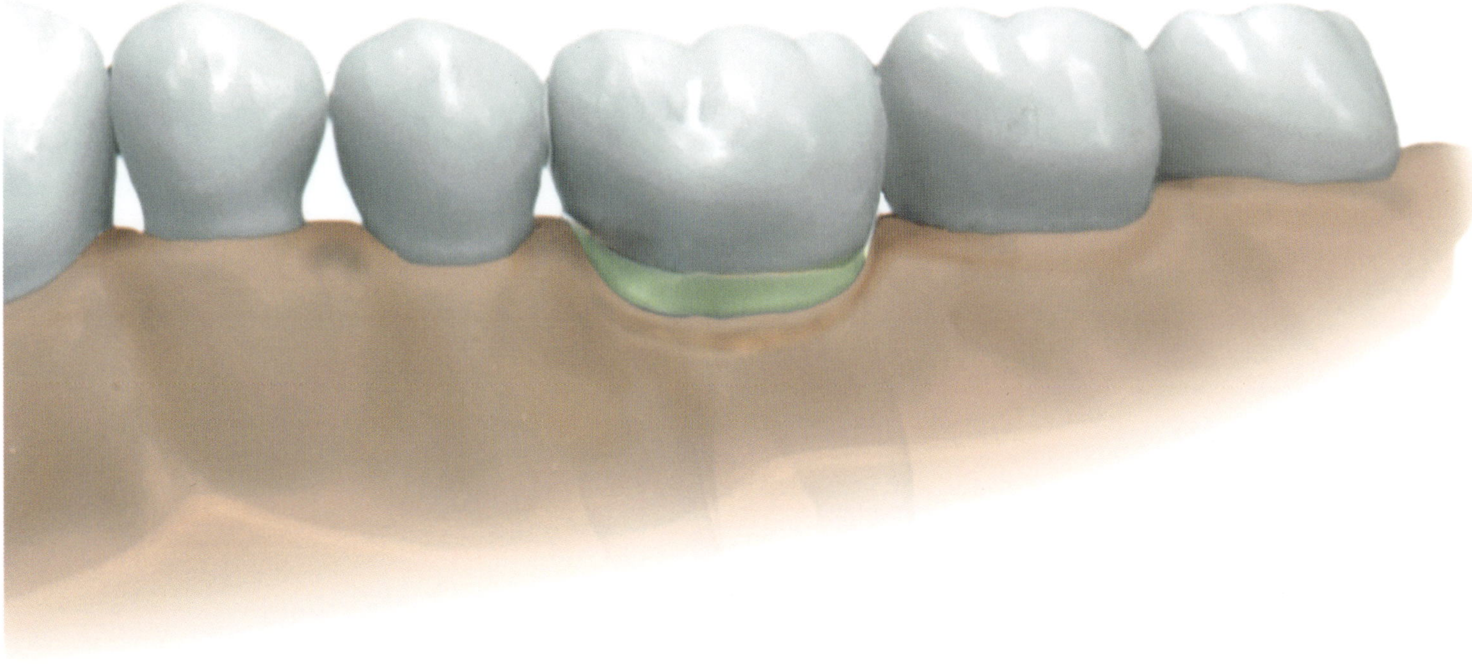

The surgery aims to lower the gingival and bony margin to access the submerged portion of the caries, in order to perform an adequate filling and relocate the tissues in apical position.

BONE GRAFT WITH MEMBRANE

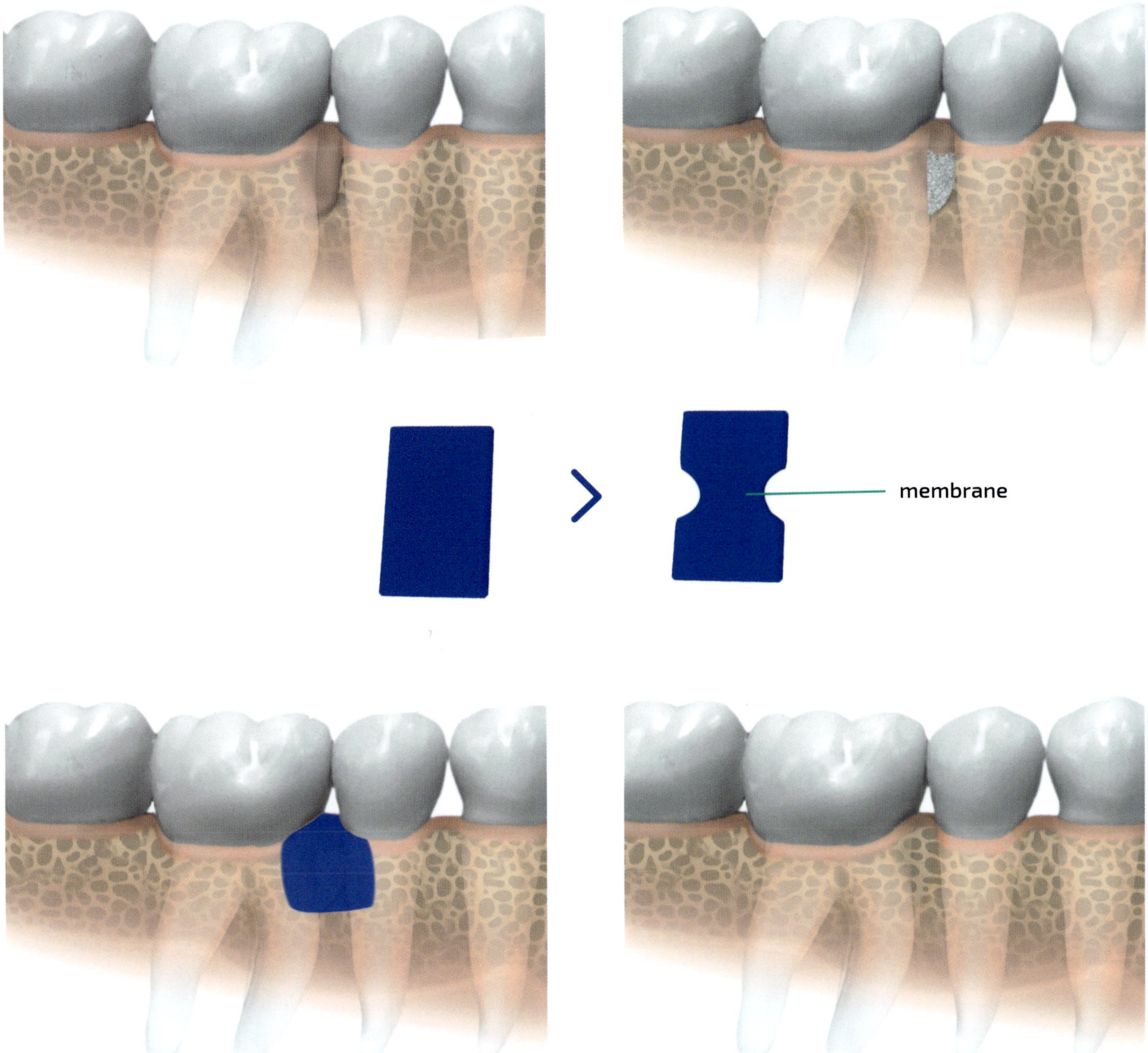

The surgery aims to correct the bone defect through the aid of autologous or heterologous bone substitutes and a resorbable or nonresorbable membrane to protect the graft.

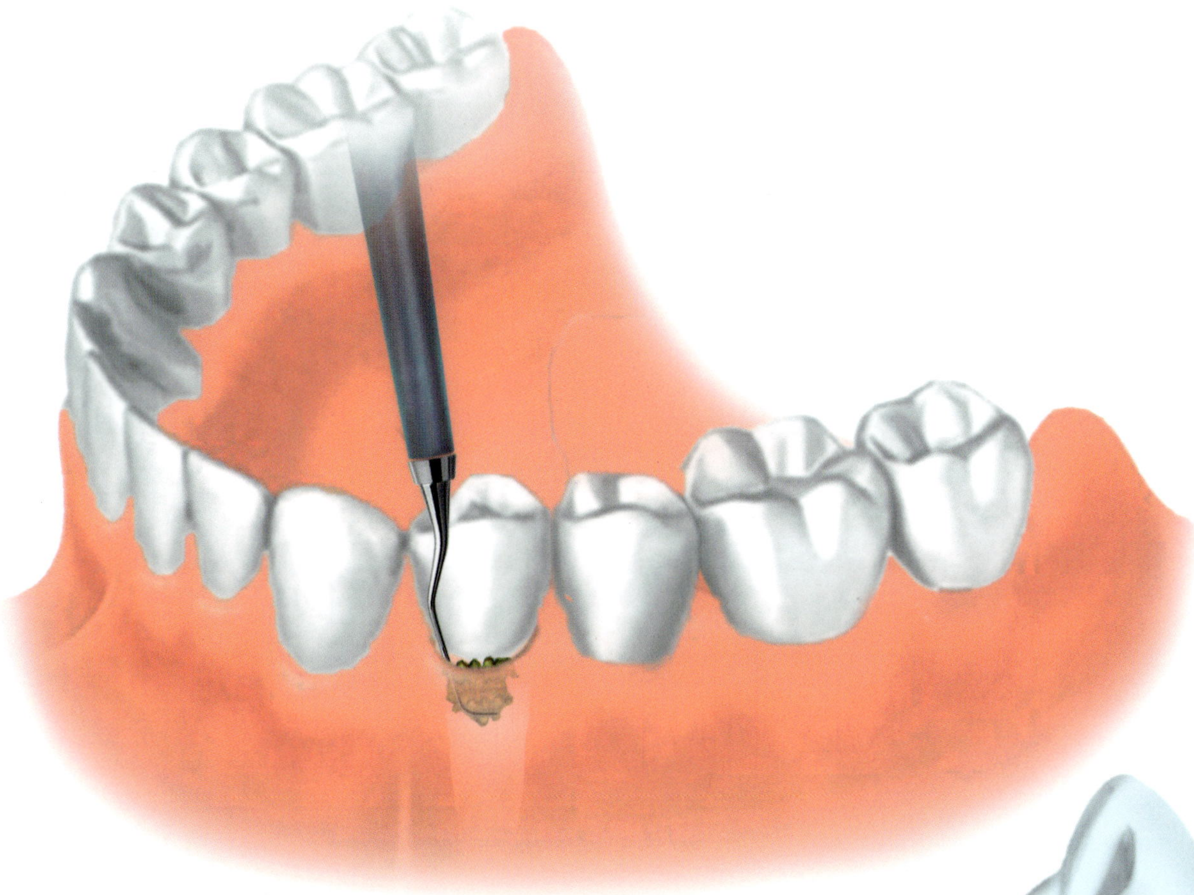

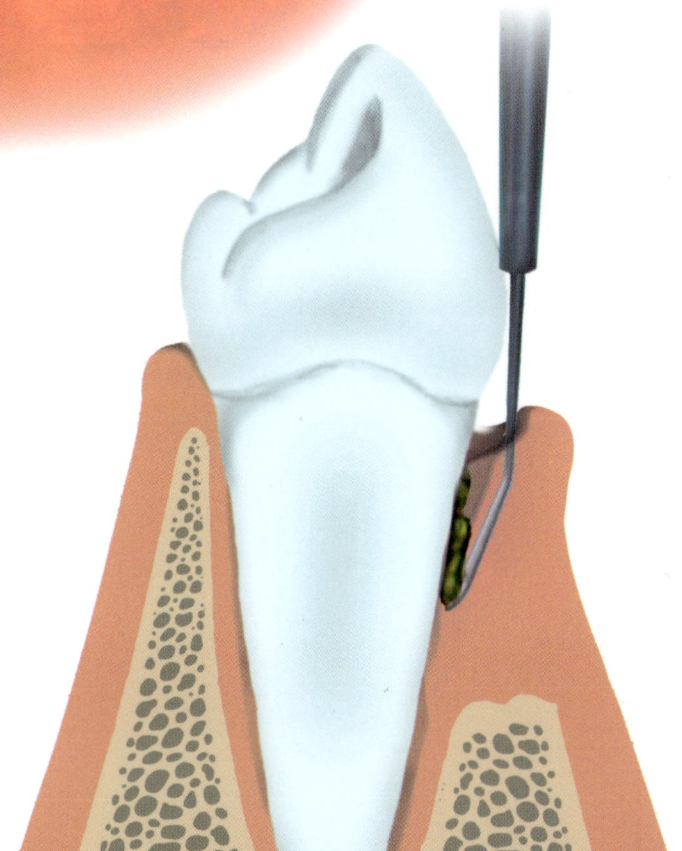

Non-surgical removal of calculus along the root surface of a tooth, within a periodontal pocket.

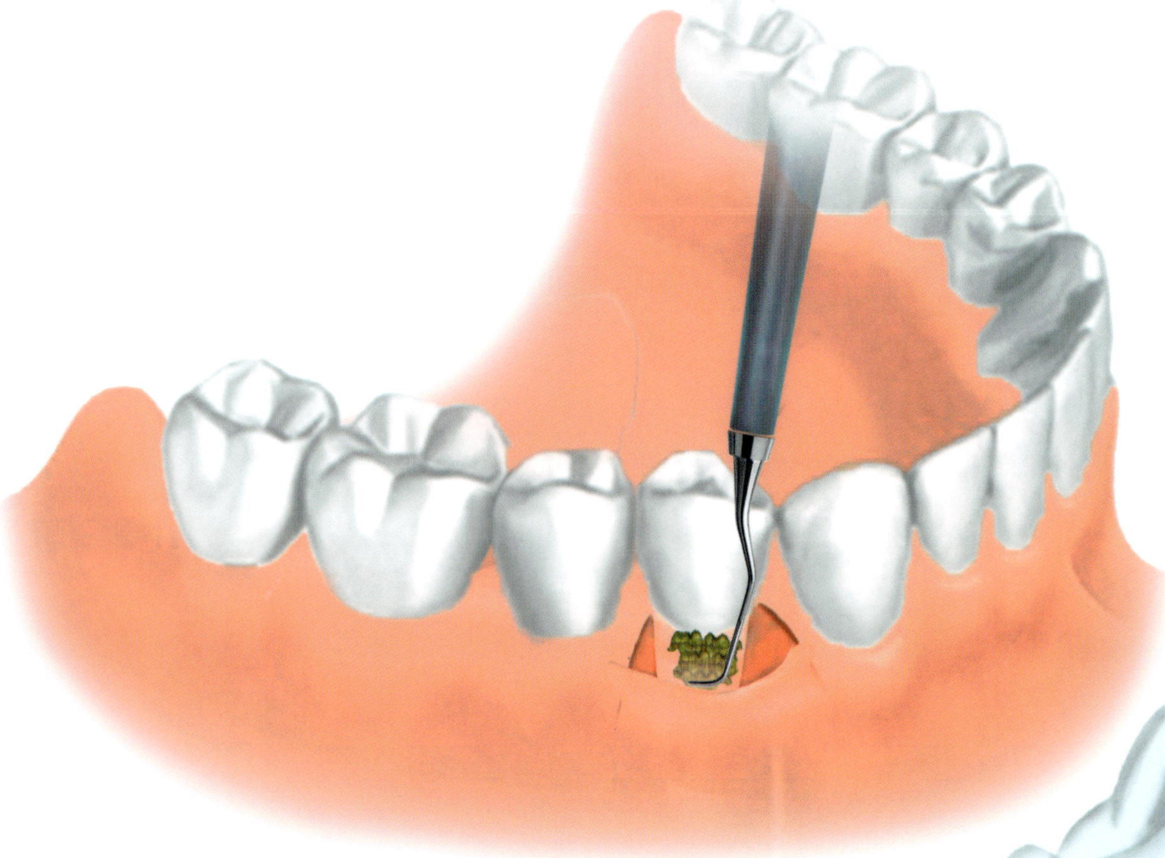

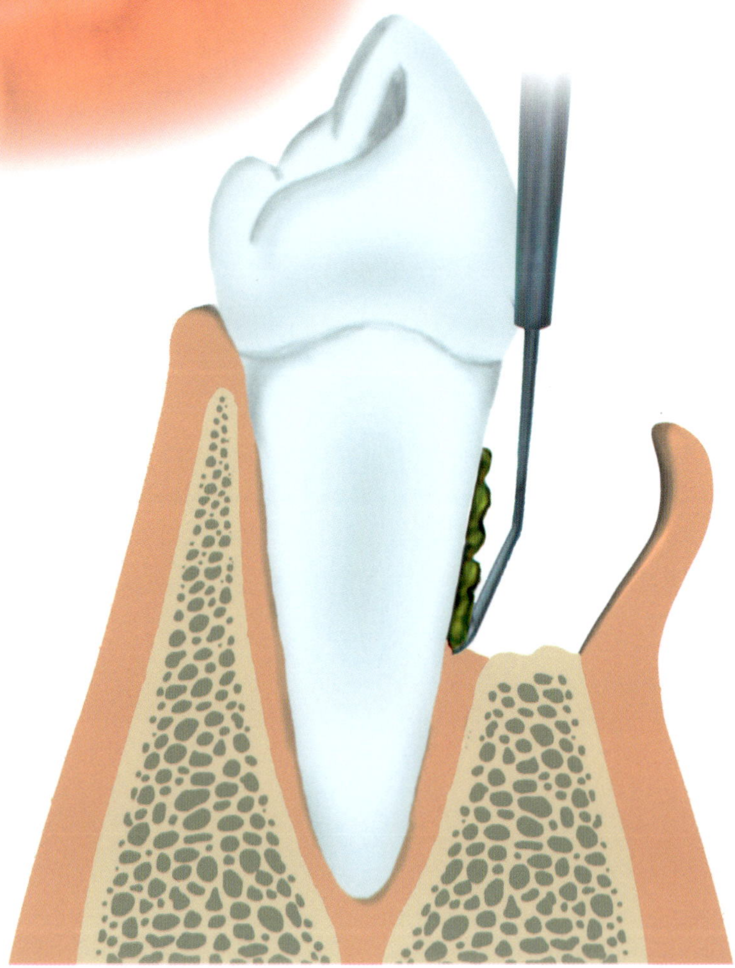

Removal of calculus along the root surface of a tooth, which involves the opening of a surgical flap.

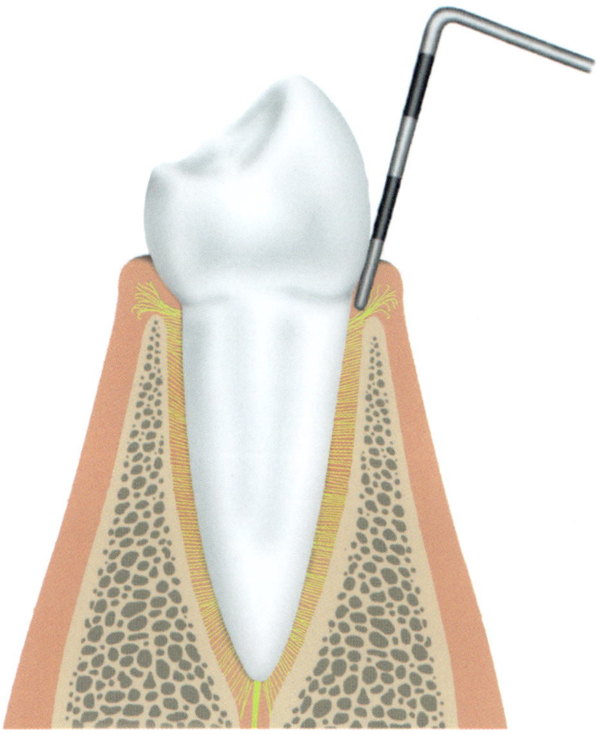

periodontal health

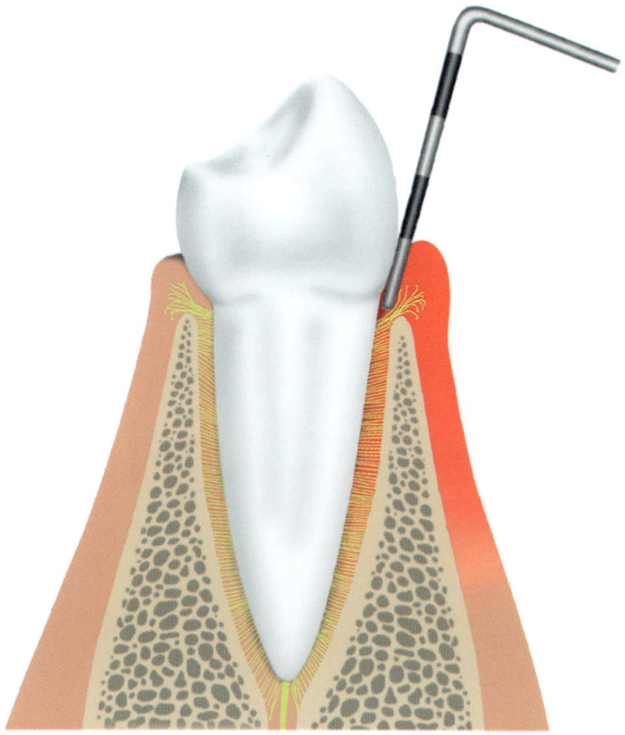

gingivitis

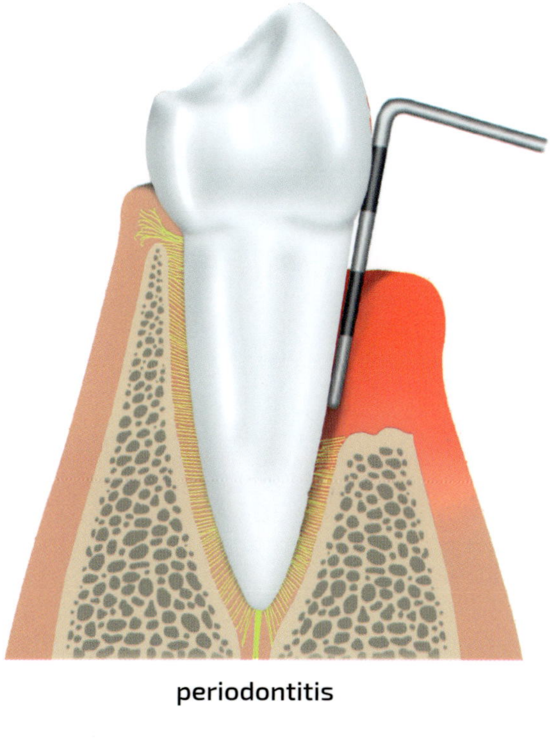

periodontitis

Sequence of clinical pictures leading to the onset of periodontal disease, which is triggered by a state of gingivitis.

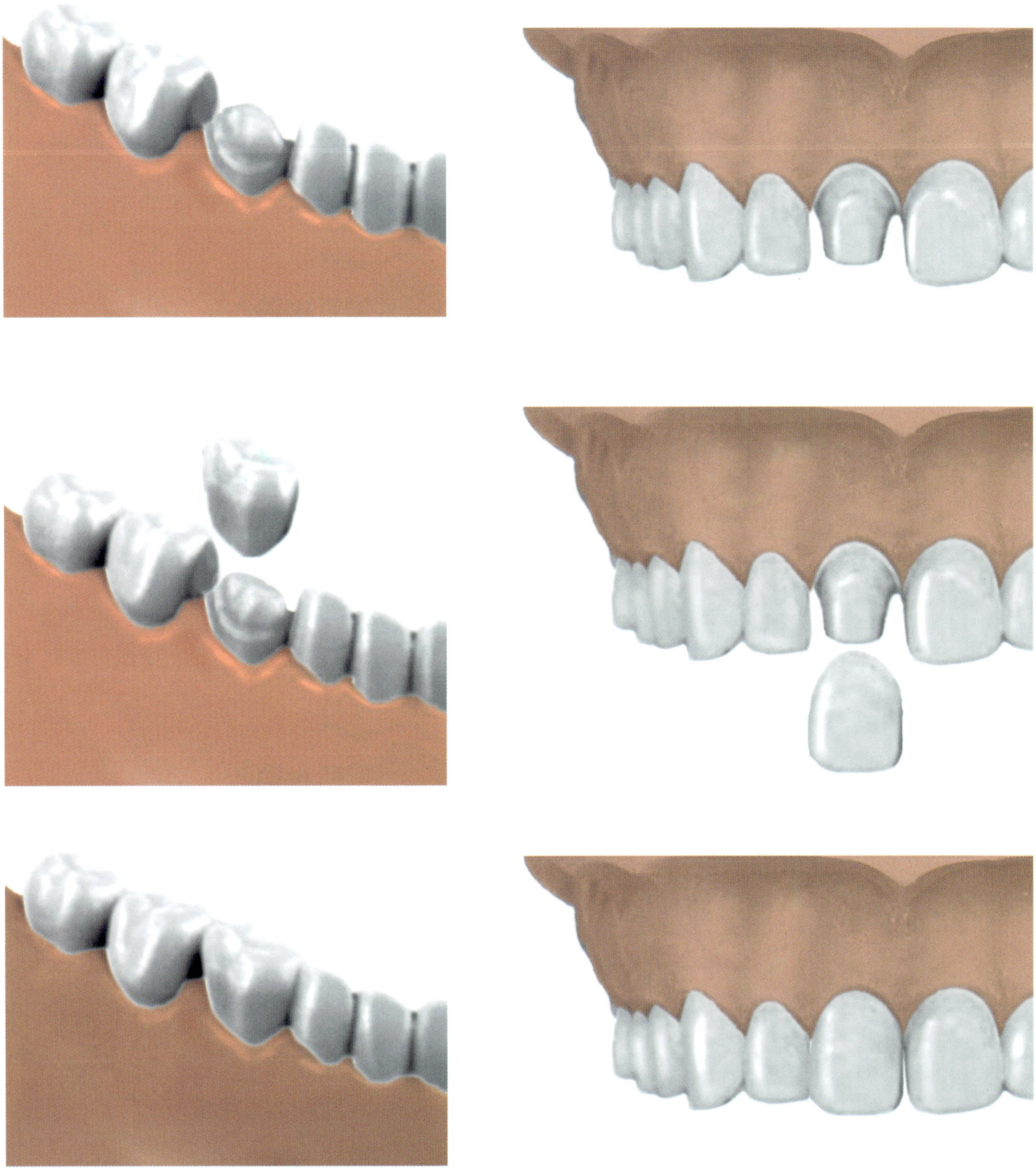

The treatment involves the tooth filing so that a prosthetic crown is cemented on it. It can be preceded by an endodontic treatment and/or direct or indirect reconstruction.

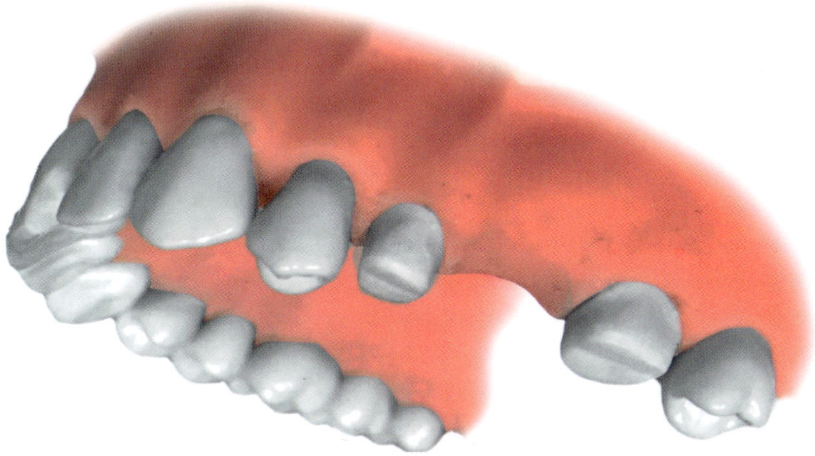

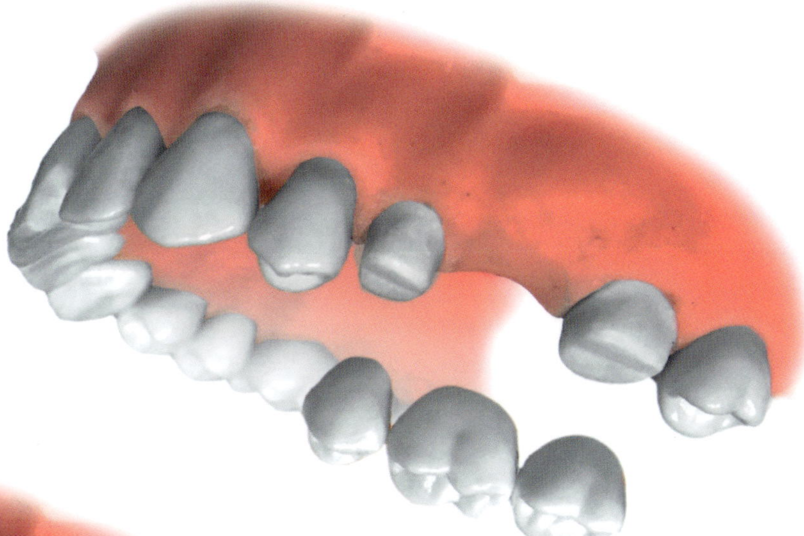

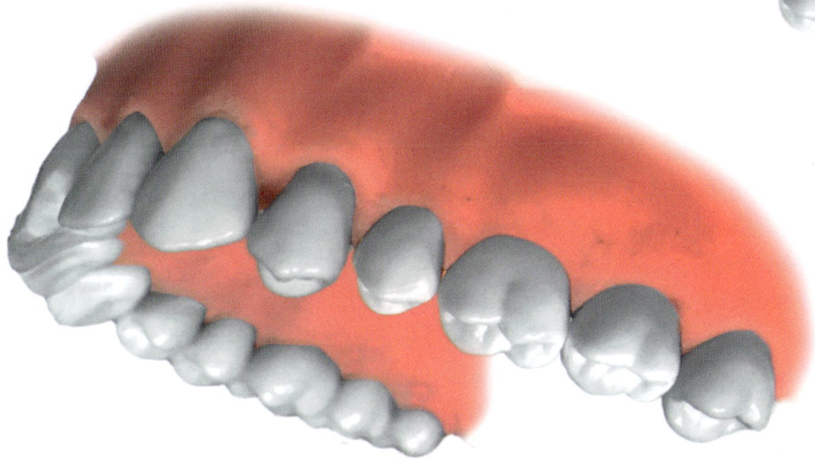

The treatment involves the teeth filing so that a structure of three prosthetic crowns is cemented on them. After their filing, they will become prosthetic abutments. It can be preceded by an endodontic treatment and/or direct or indirect reconstruction.

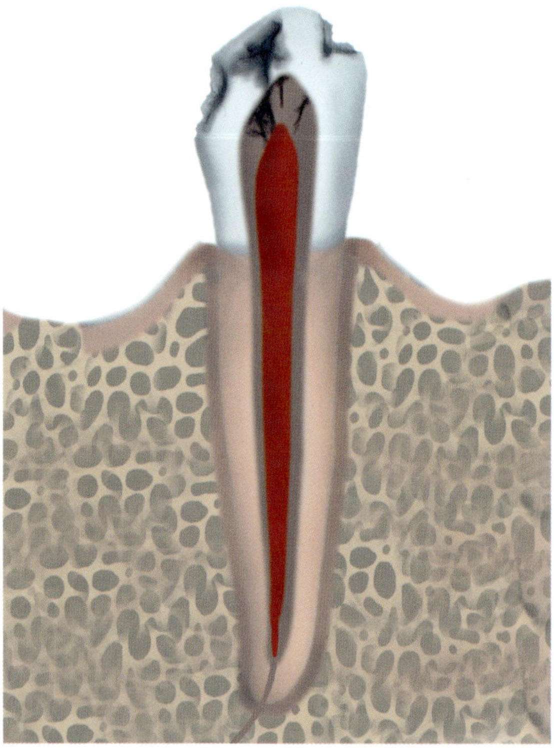

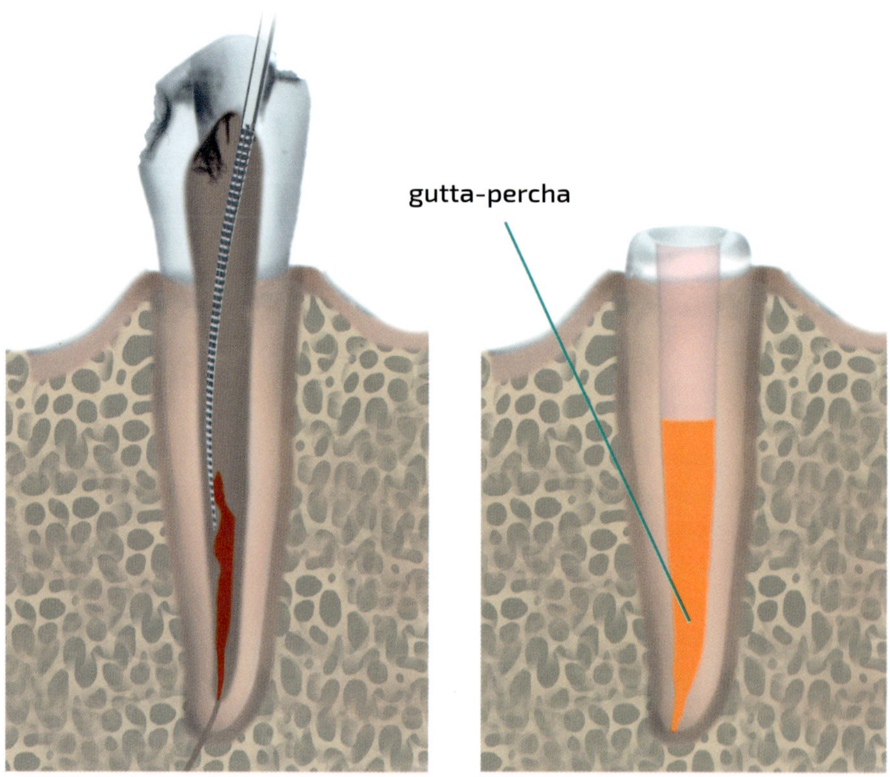

The condition of the tooth does not allow its full functional restoration with conservative therapy alone. After endodontic therapy it will be necessary to insert a pin abutment inside the canal, on which a prosthetic crown will later be cemented.

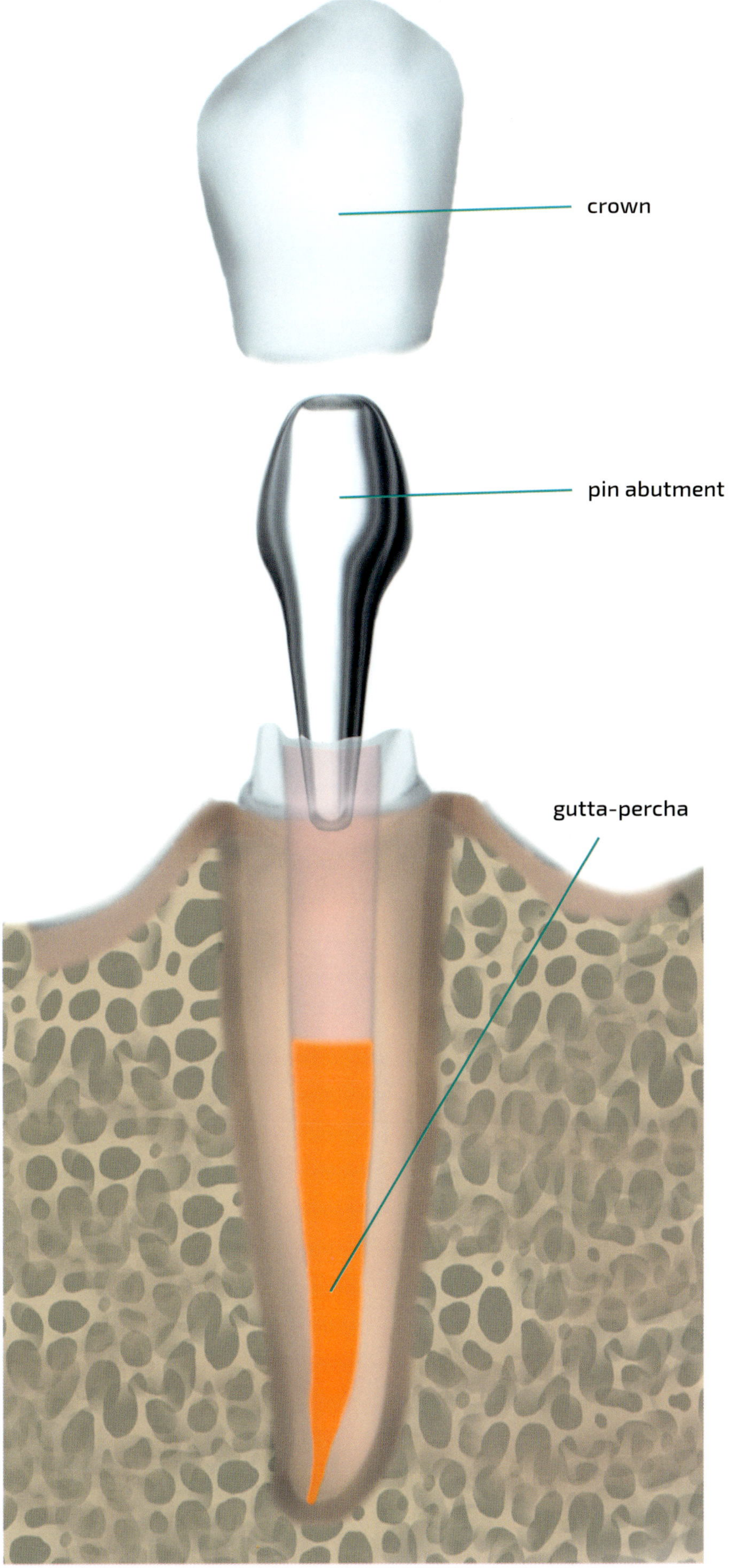
crown
pin abutment
gutta-percha

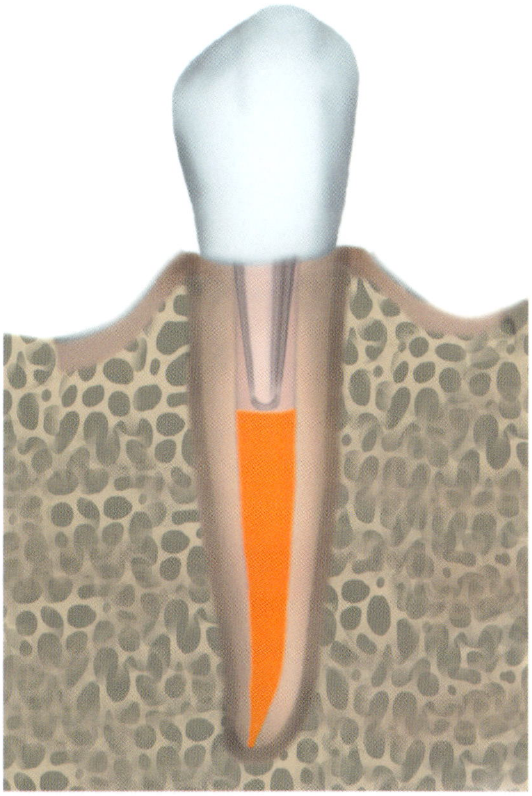

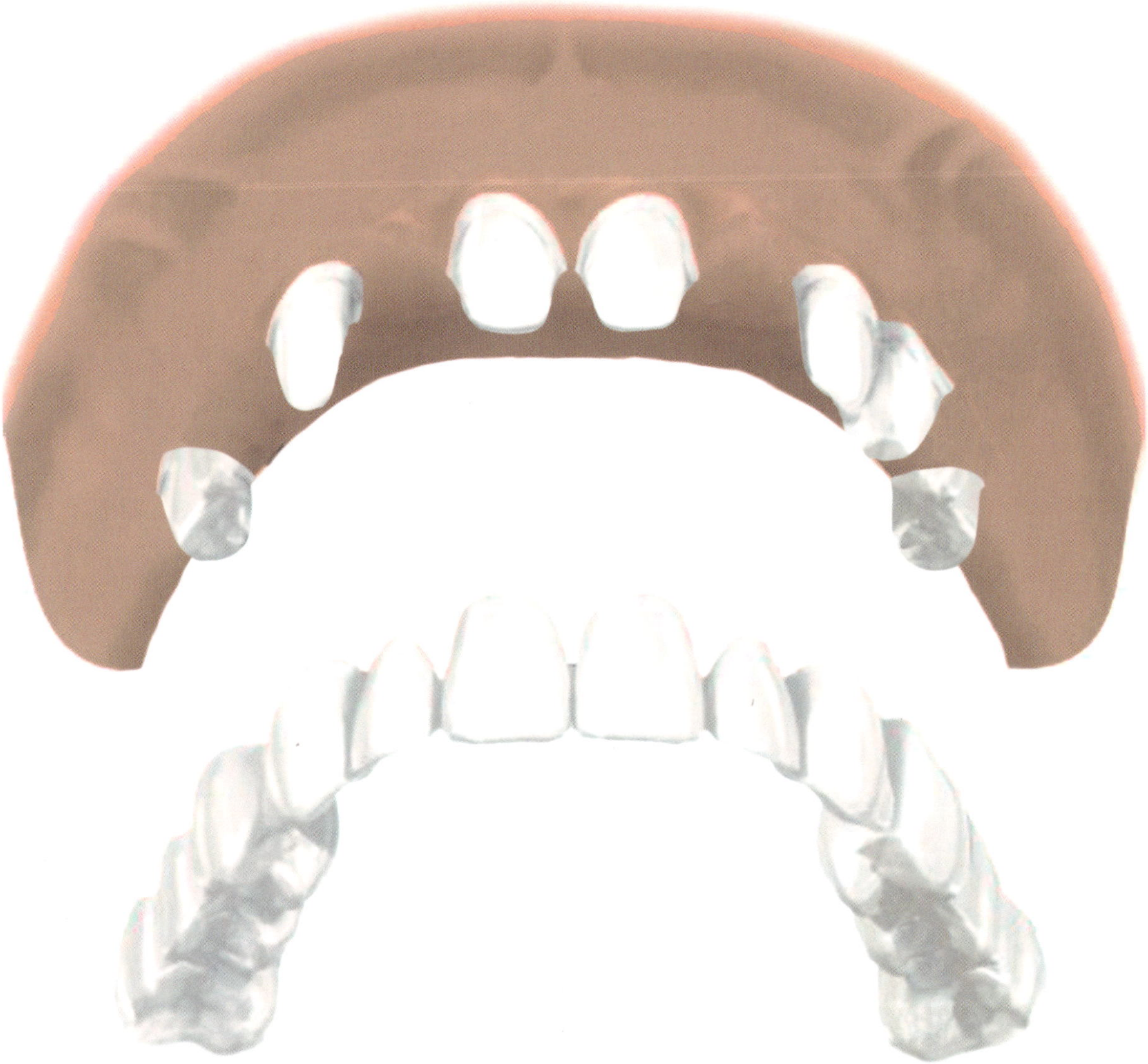

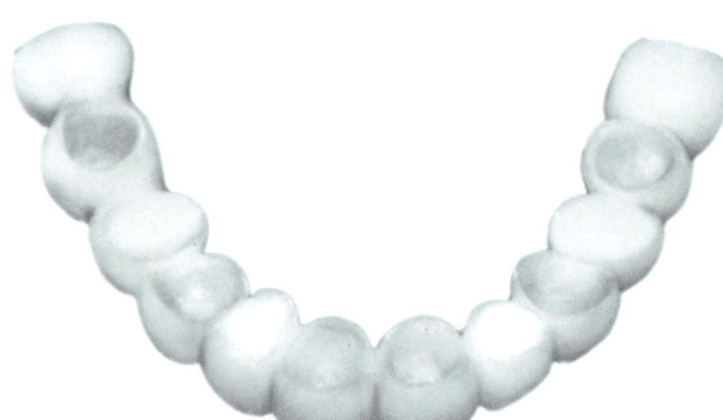

Prosthetic rehabilitation of an entire arch carried out following the preparation of the residual elements and a subsequent impression taking, from which the prosthetic product will be made in the laboratory.

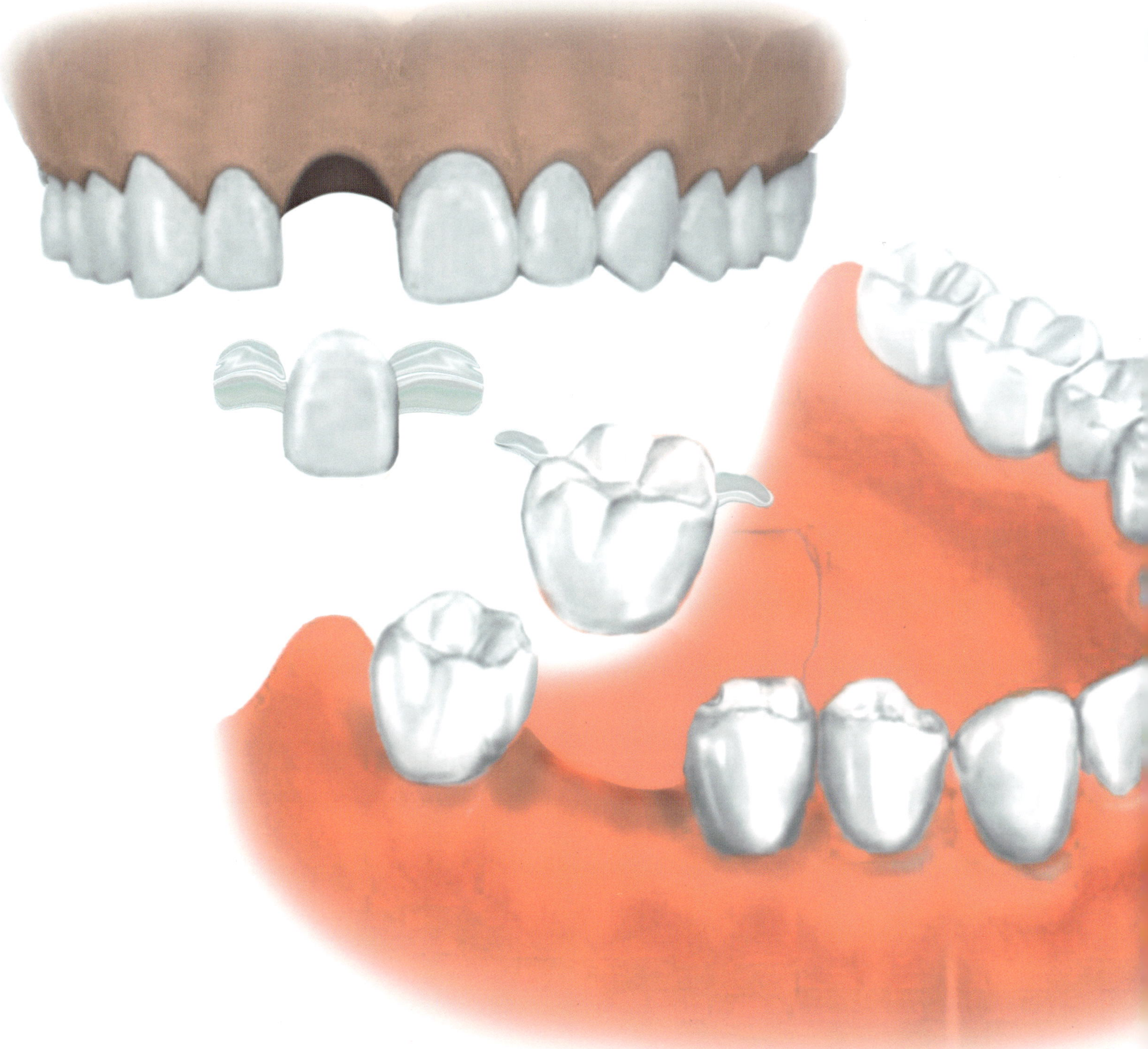

Replacement of a single tooth through a prosthesis with lateral or occlusal flaps, which will be cemented on the elements adjacent to the missing element.

ENDODONTIC THERAPY SINGLE-ROOTED TOOTH

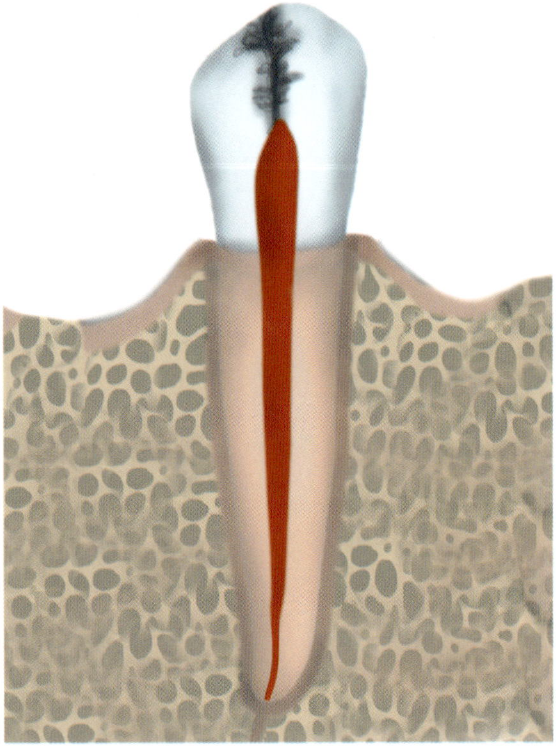

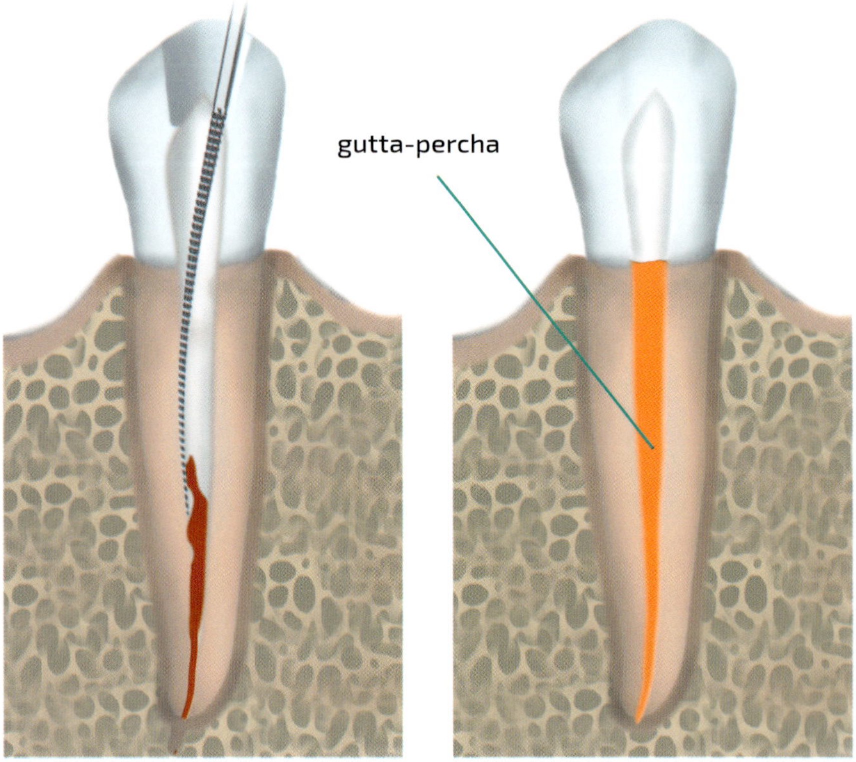

Treatment is necessary when the tooth has penetrating caries, with pulpitis or pulp necrosis. It involves the removal of the dental pulp, the cleaning and shaping of the canals and their closure at the apex with gutta-percha.

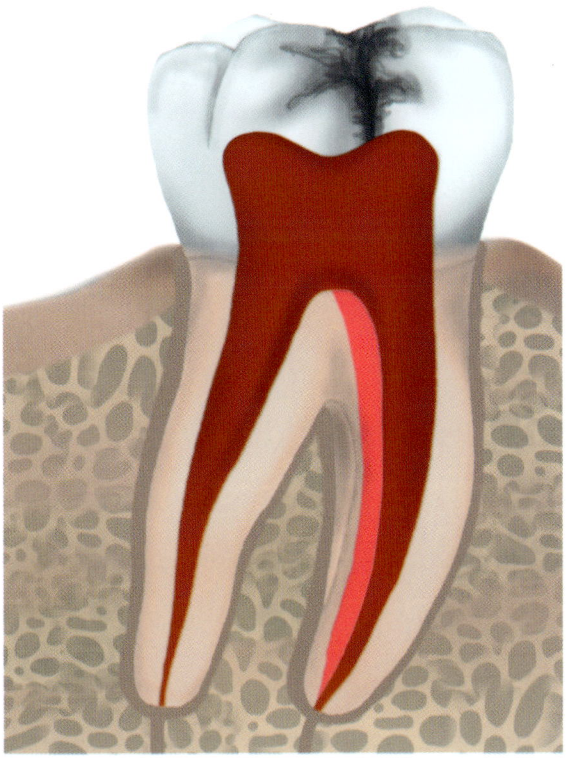

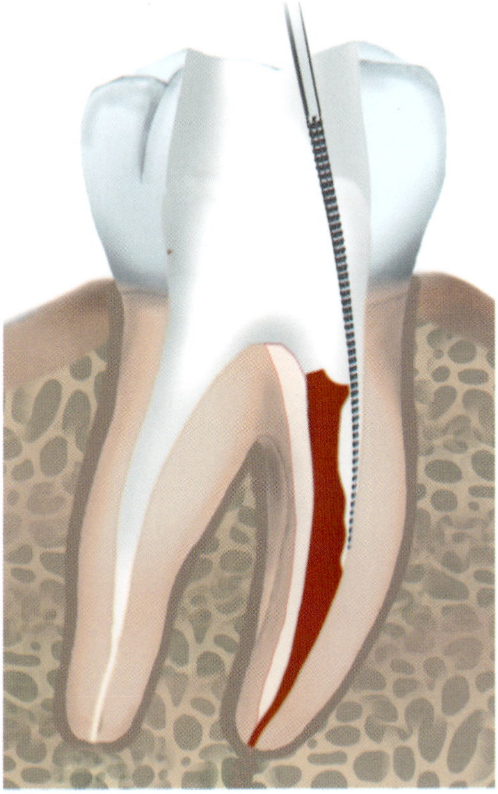

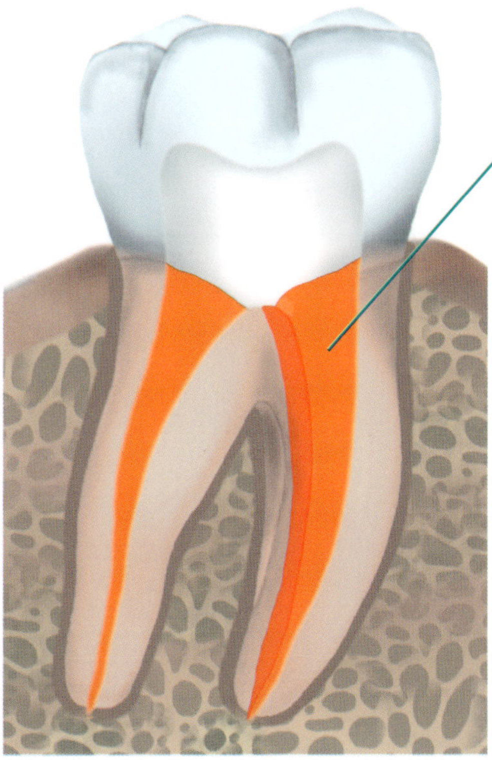
gutta-percha

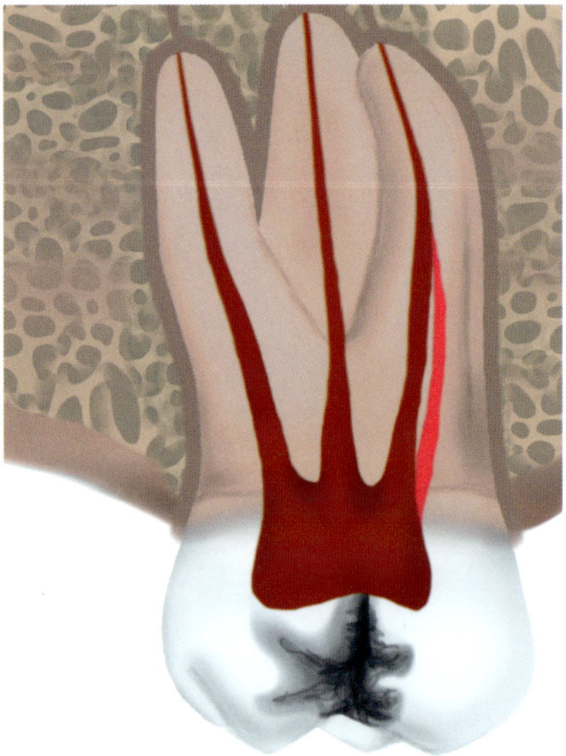

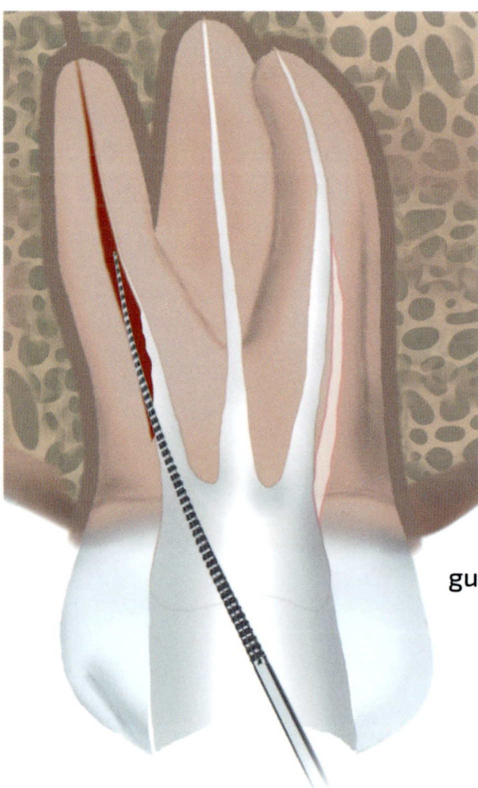

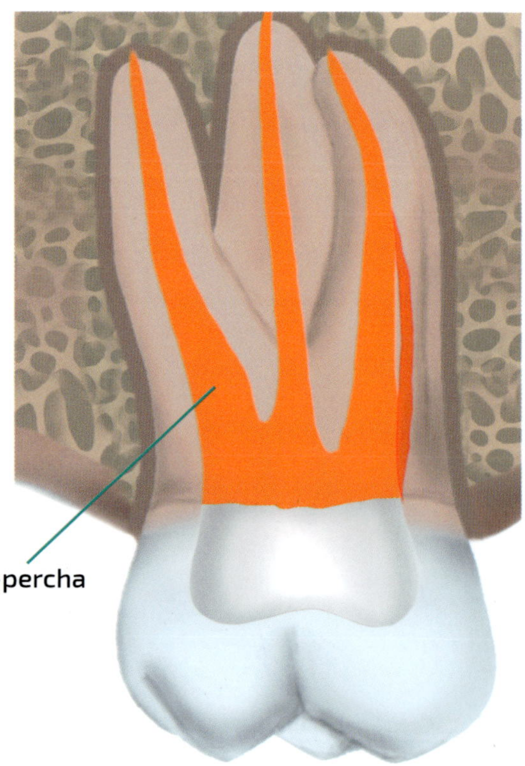

Treatment is necessary when the tooth has penetrating caries, with pulpitis or pulp necrosis. It involves the removal of the dental pulp, the cleaning and shaping of the canals and their closure at the apex with gutta-percha.

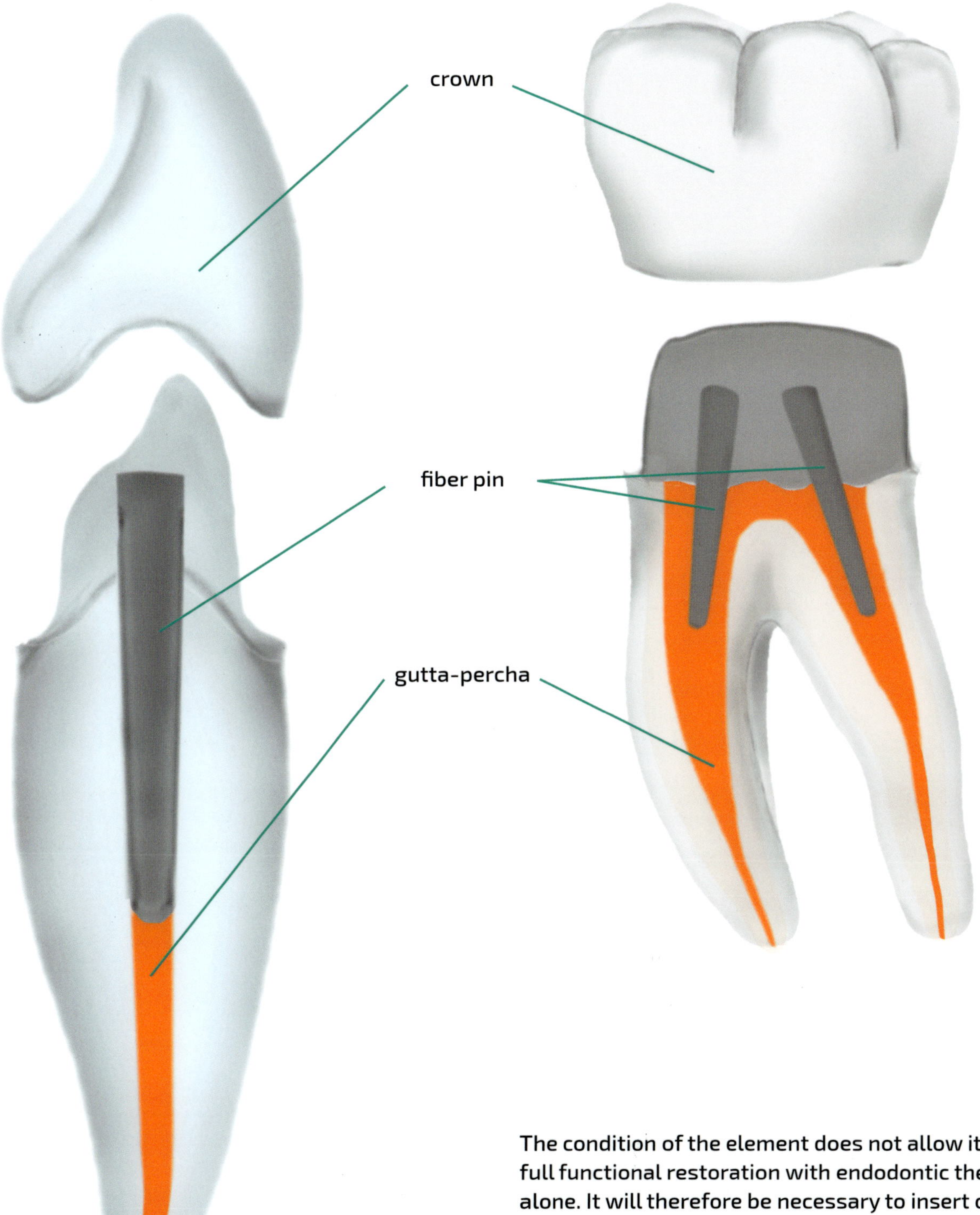

The condition of the element does not allow its full functional restoration with endodontic therapy alone. It will therefore be necessary to insert one or more carbon or glass fiber pins inside the canal, around which an abutment will be made on which a prosthetic crown will be cemented.

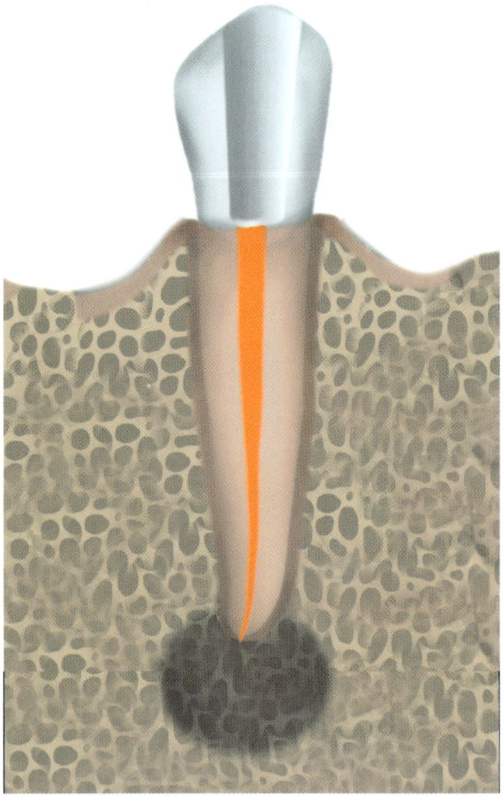

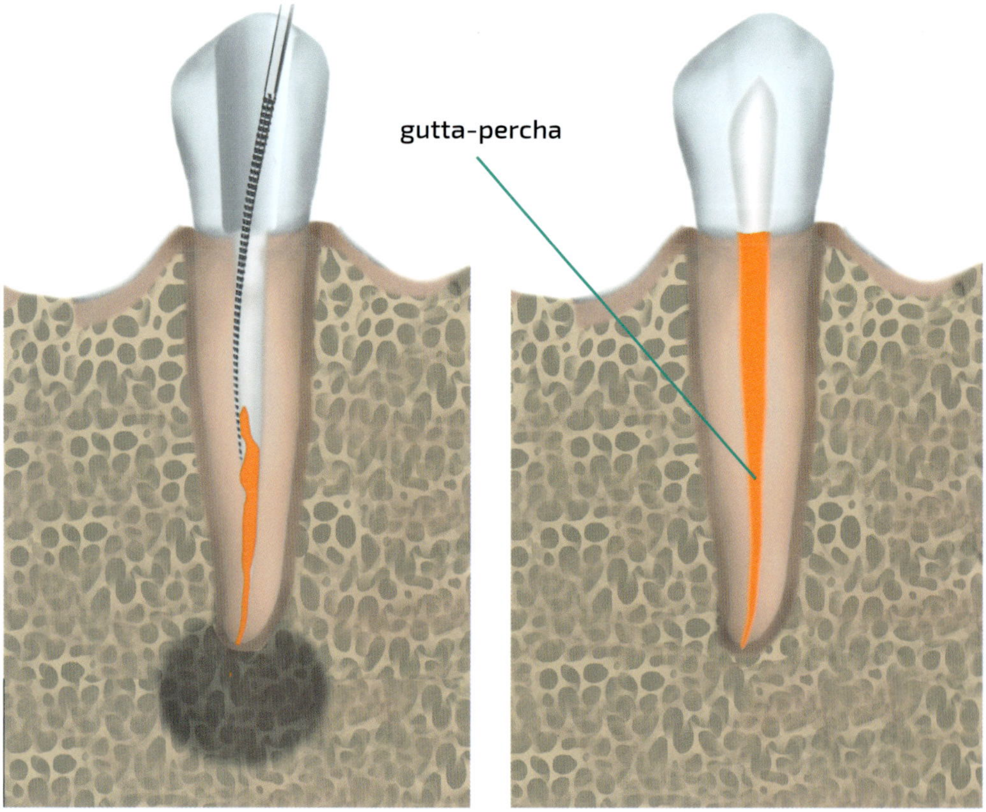

The treatment allows to intervene again on a previously devitalized tooth, in which a periapical lesion is radiographically visible. The gutta-percha will be removed and the tooth will undergo again endodontic treatment.

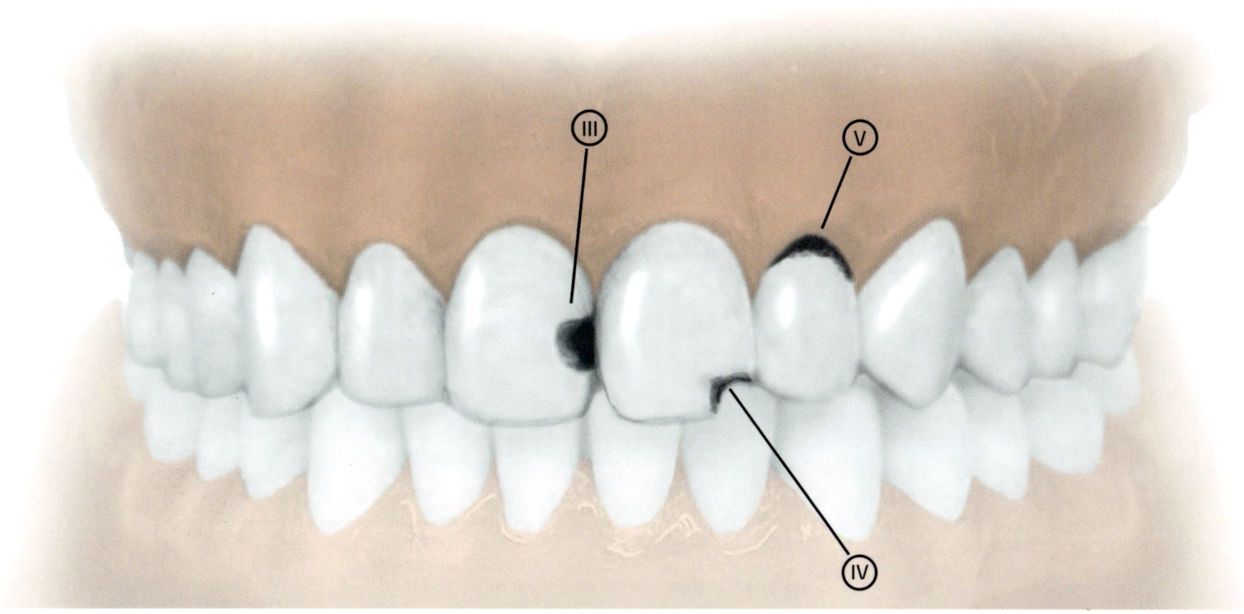

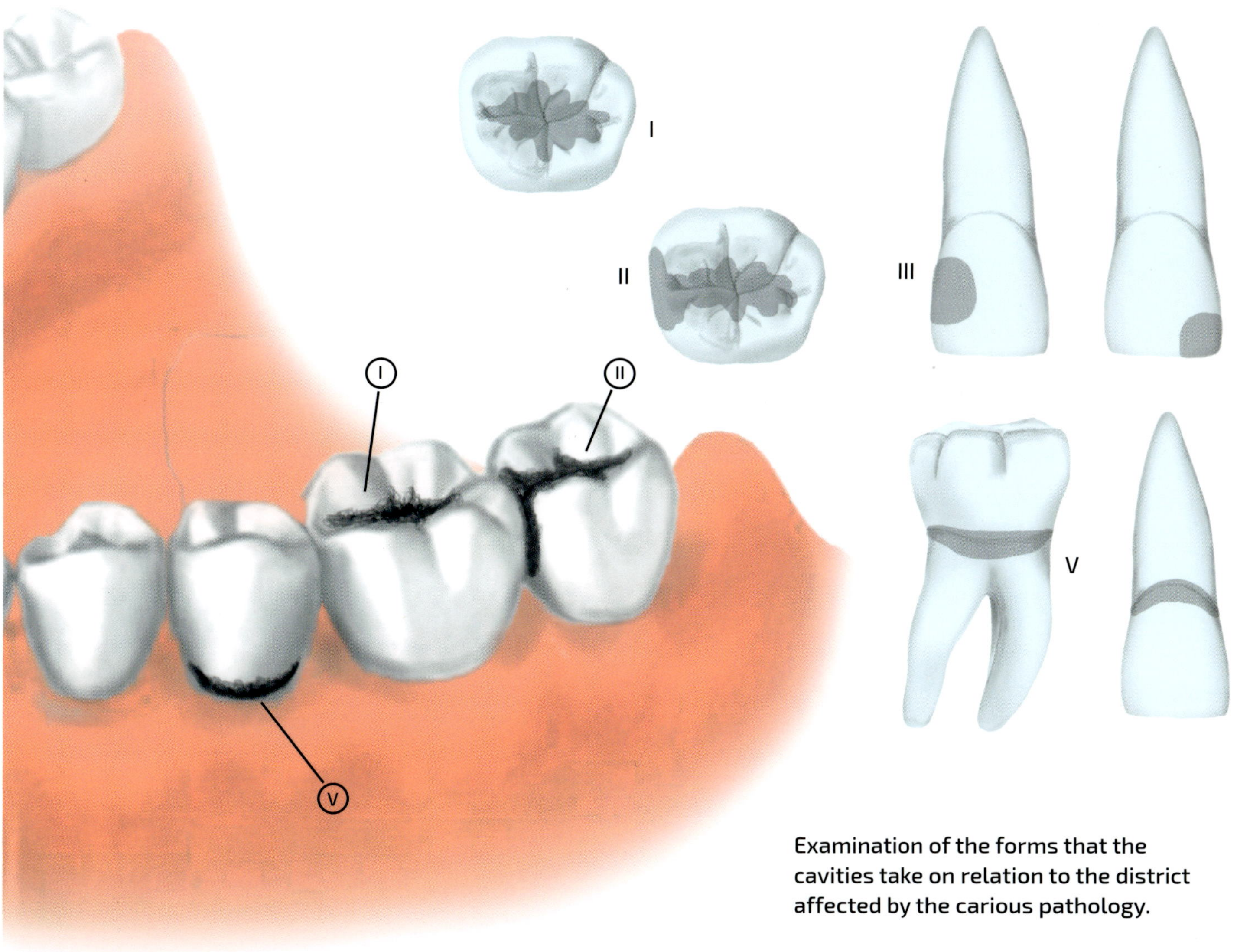

Examination of the forms that the cavities take on relation to the district affected by the carious pathology.

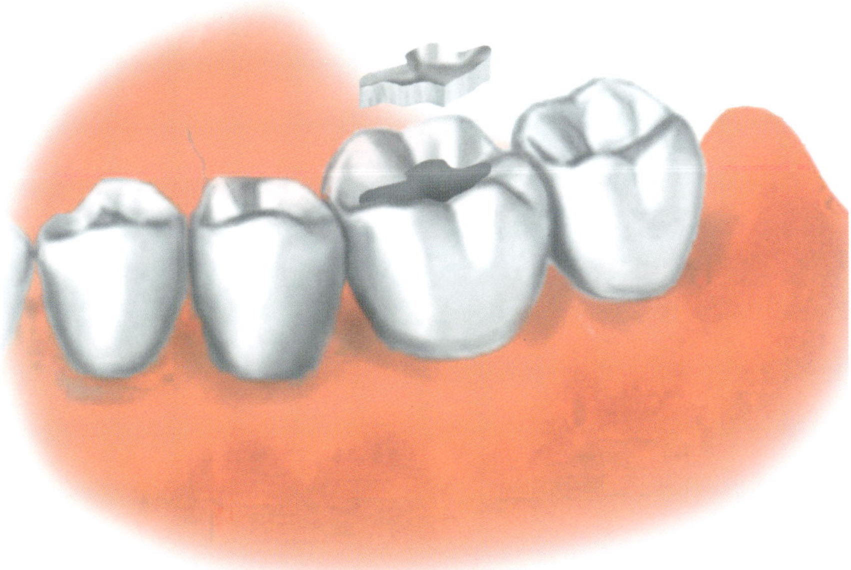

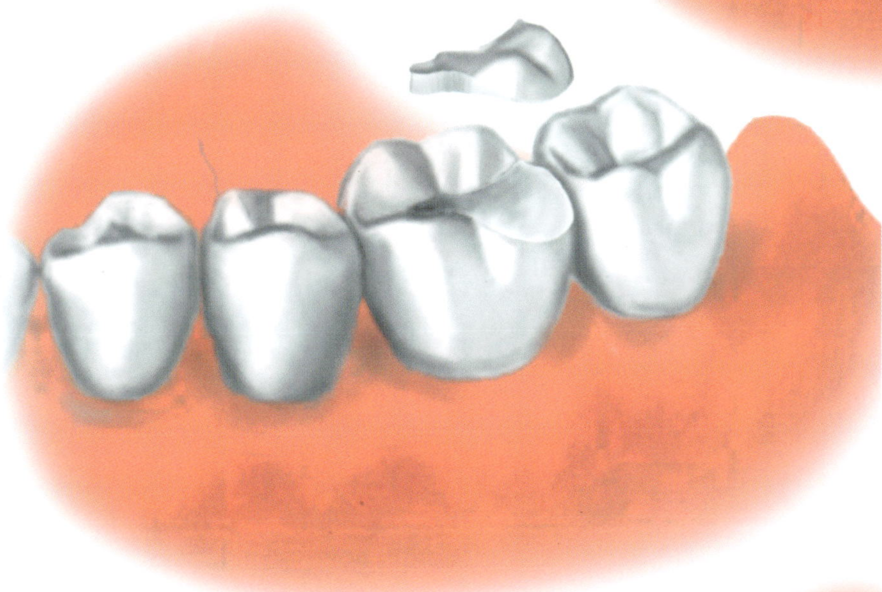

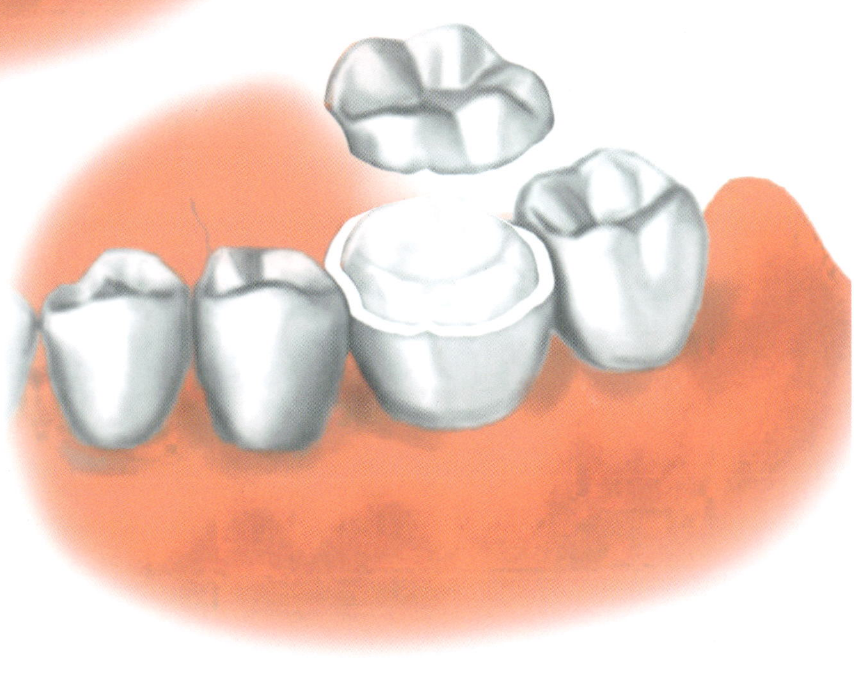

Aesthetic-functional restoration of a tooth, involving the cementation of a small prosthetic product made in the laboratory after preparation and impression, instead of a conservative reconstruction performed directly in the dental office.

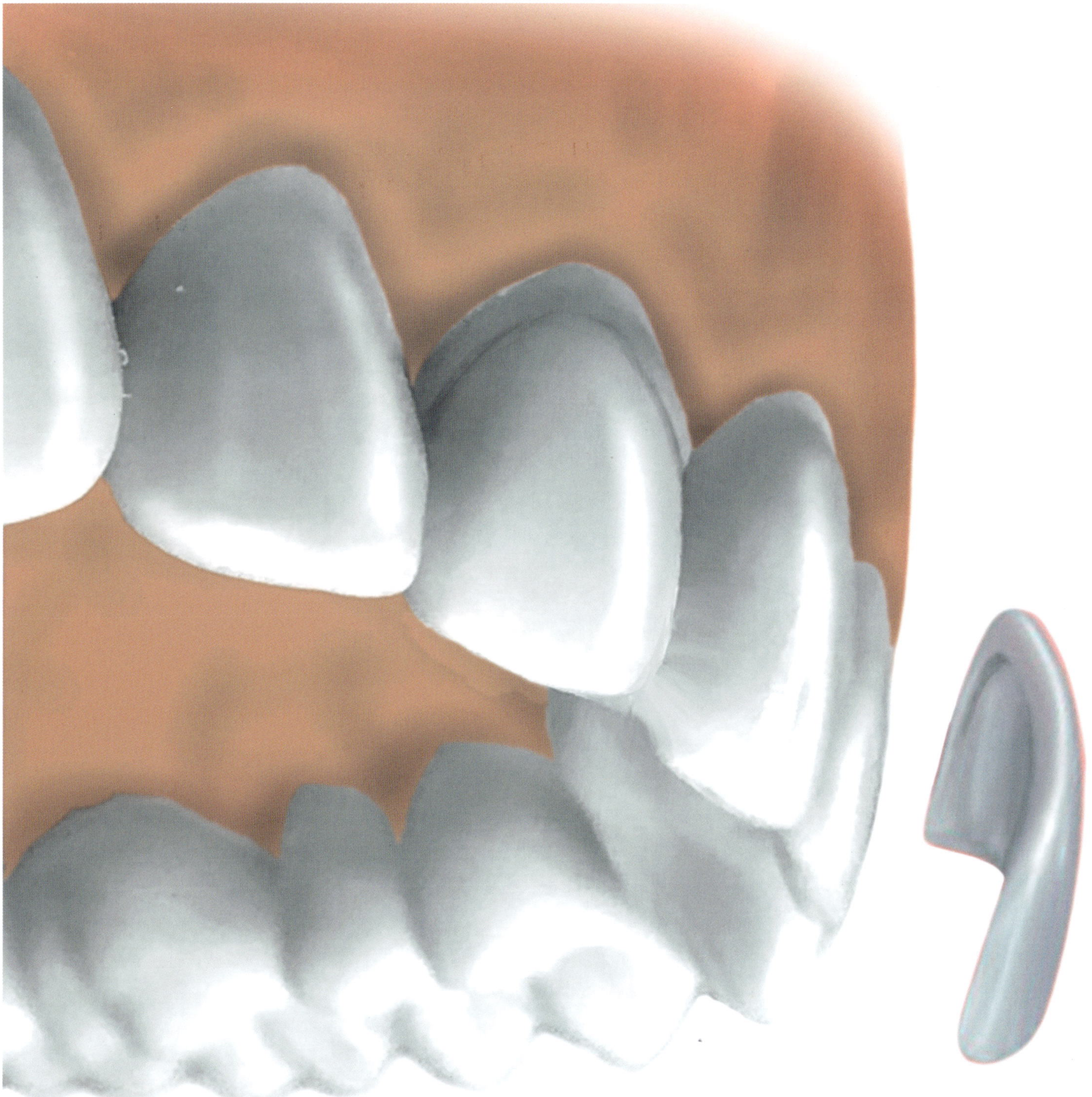

Aesthetic-functional restoration of a tooth involving the filing, limited to the vestibular side, and the subsequent cementation of the external veneer which can be made of different materials.

SKELETON WITH HOOKS ON CANINES

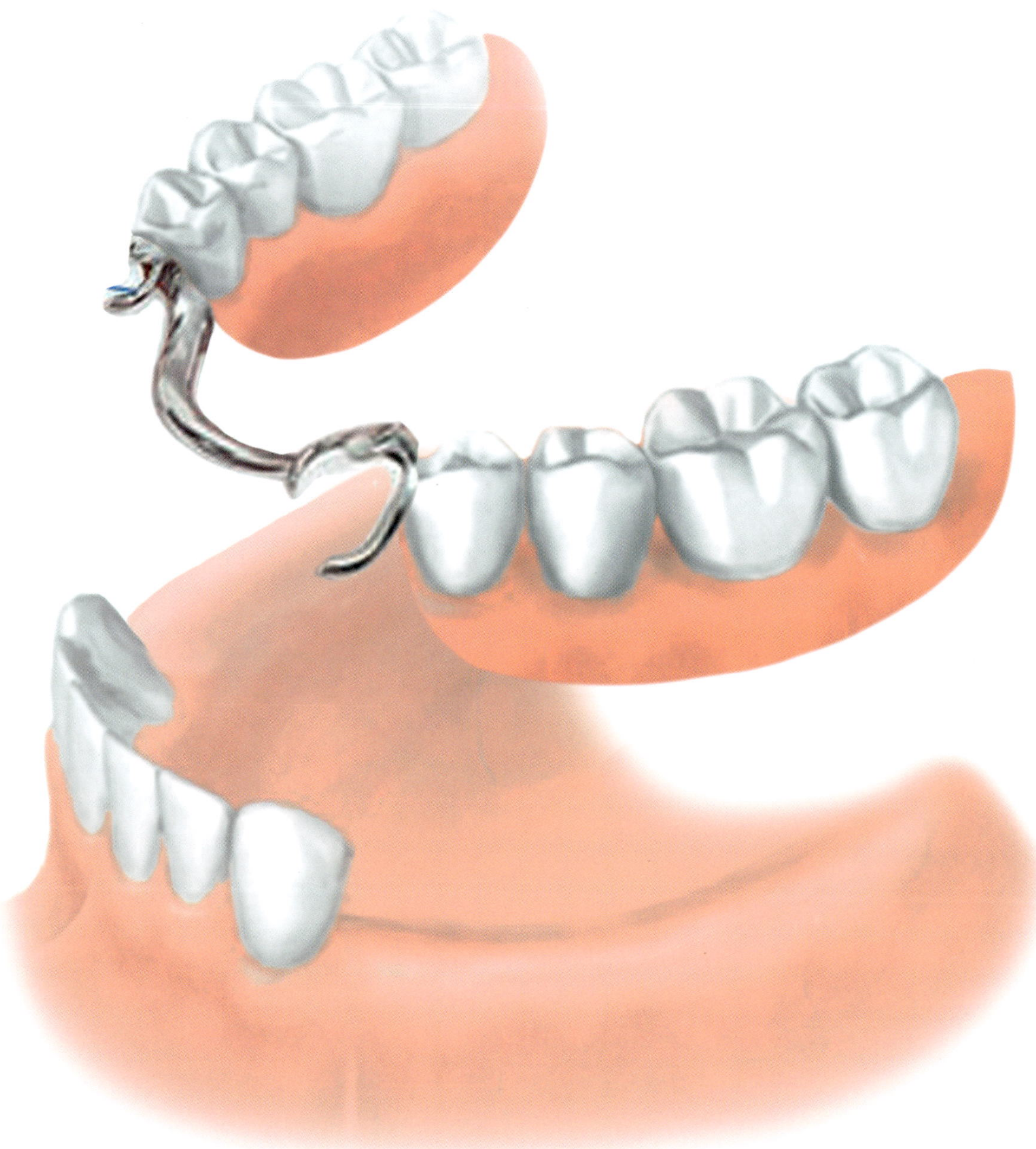

Removable prosthetic device with dentomucosal support, fixed to the teeth by retentive hooks.
In this case the artifact will be hooked to the canines.

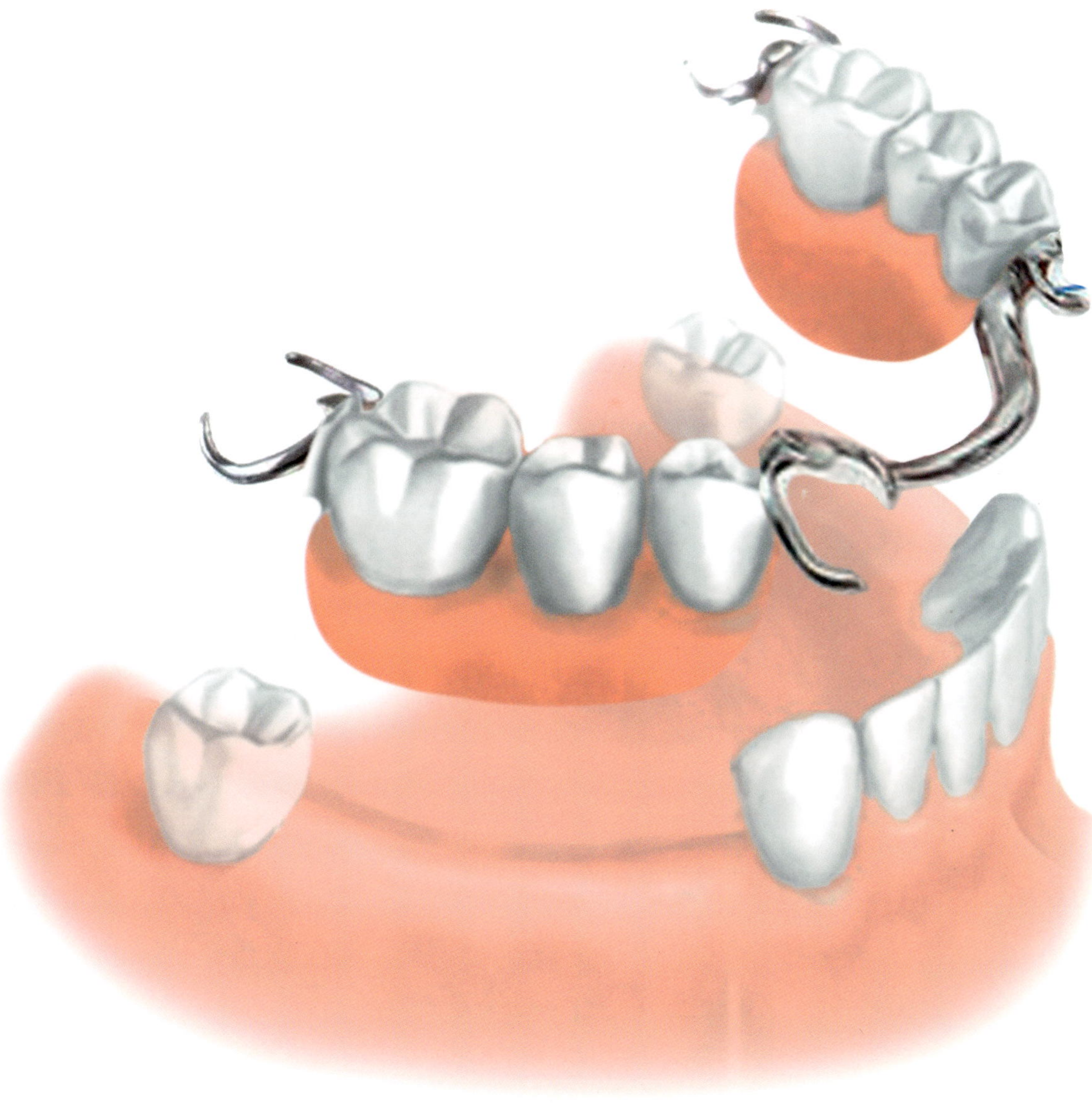

Removable prosthetic device with dentomucosal support, fixed to the teeth by retentive hooks. In this case the artifact will also be hooked to the molars.

SKELETON WITH CENTRAL LOCKING ATTACHMENTS FROM CANINE TO CANINE

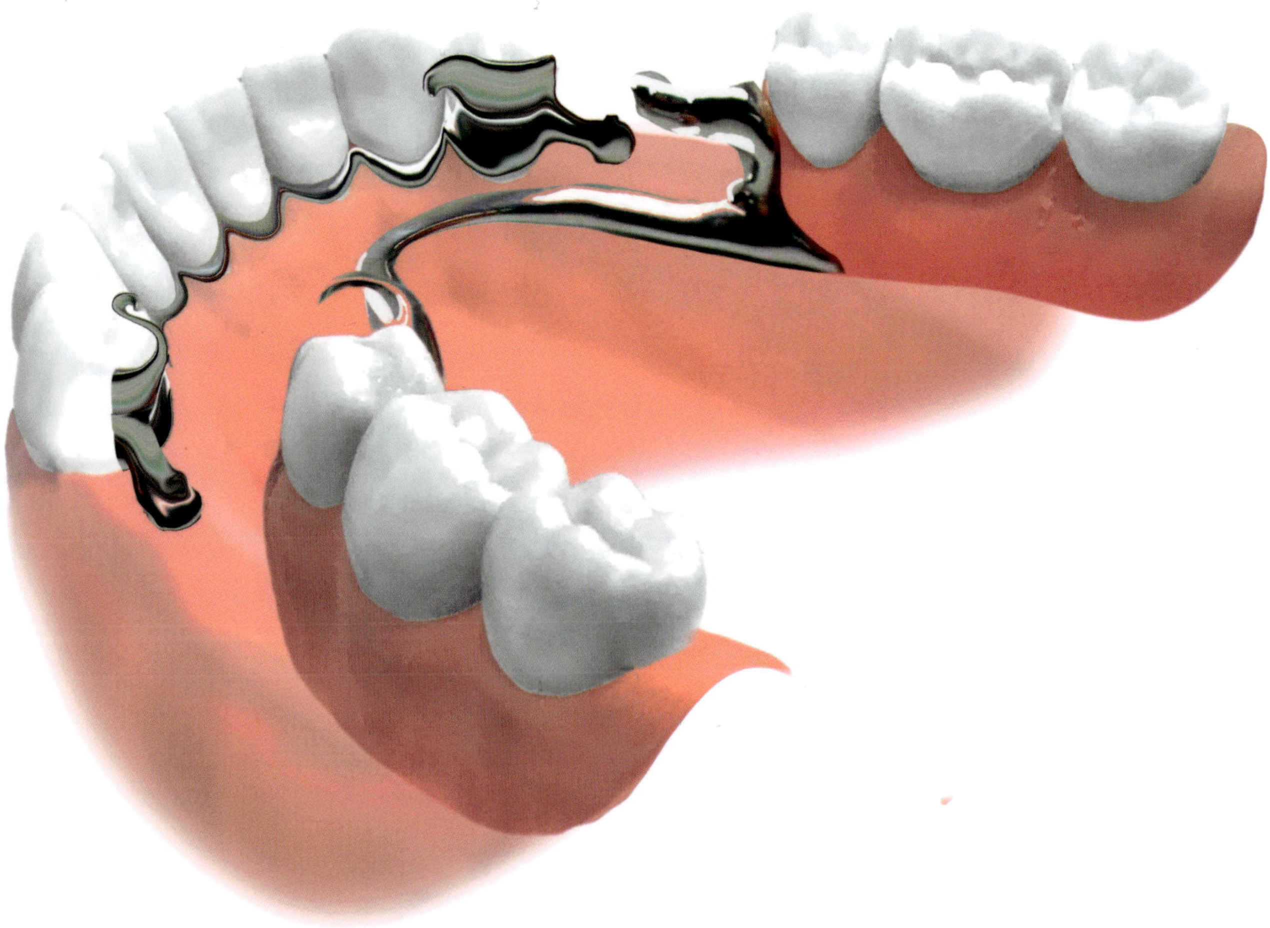

Removable prosthetic device with dentomucosal support, fixed to the teeth by means of attachments that are welded to prosthetic crowns.

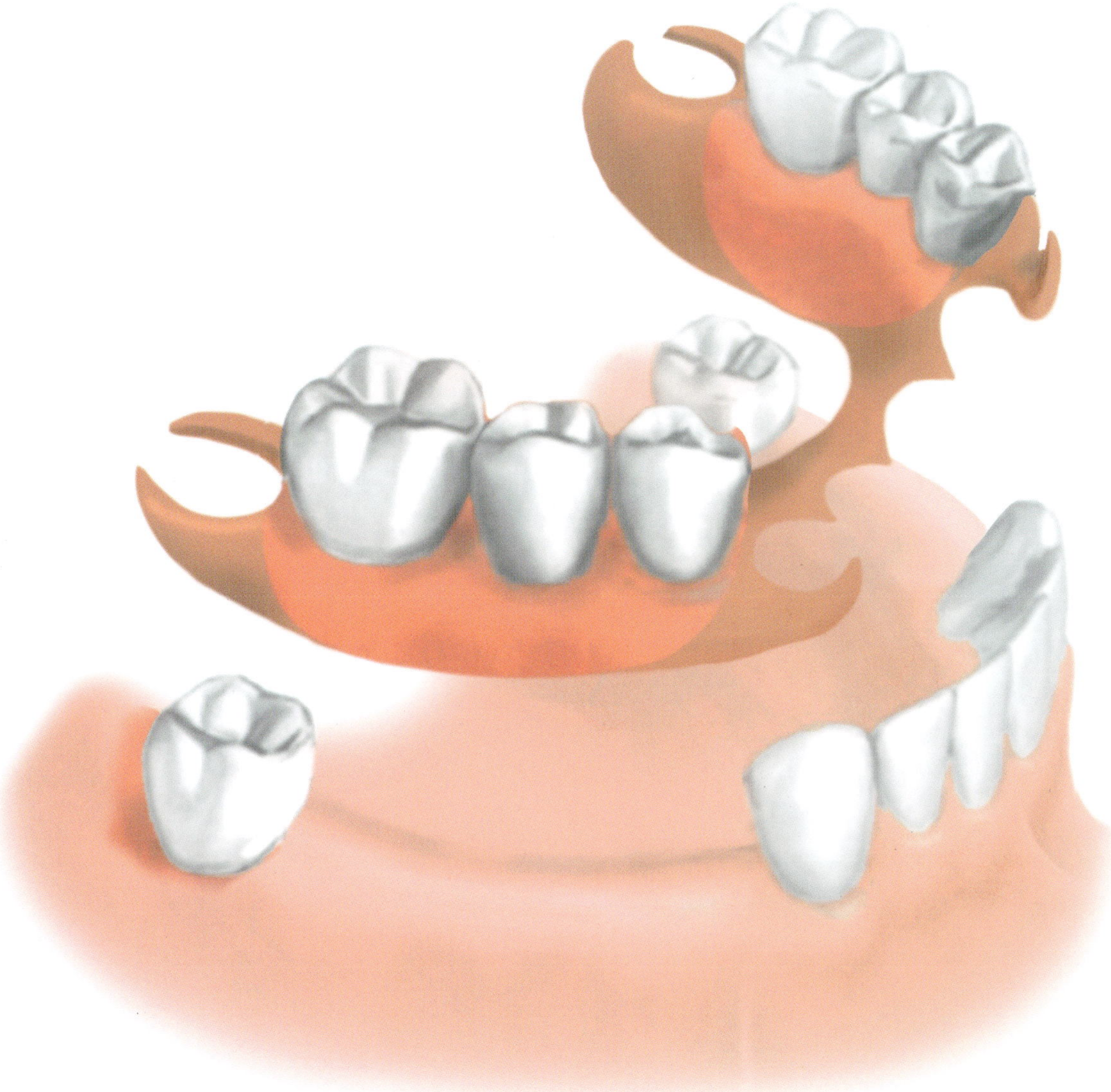

Removable prosthetic device with dentomucosal support, fixed to the teeth by means of thermoplastic nylon aesthetic hooks.

LOWER THIRD MOLAR HORIZONTAL WITH LESION OF THE SECOND MOLAR

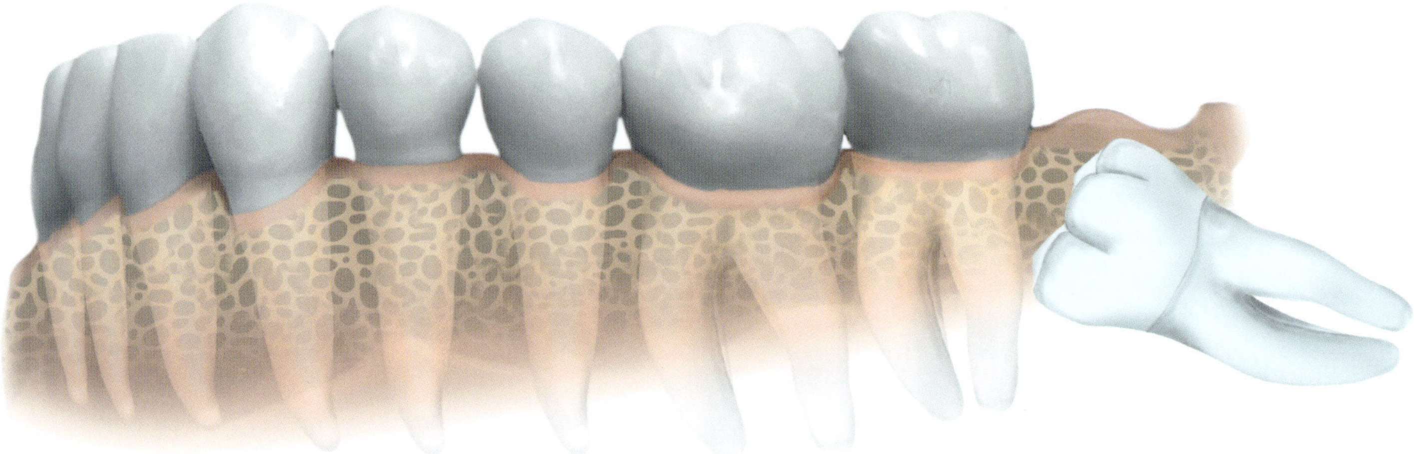

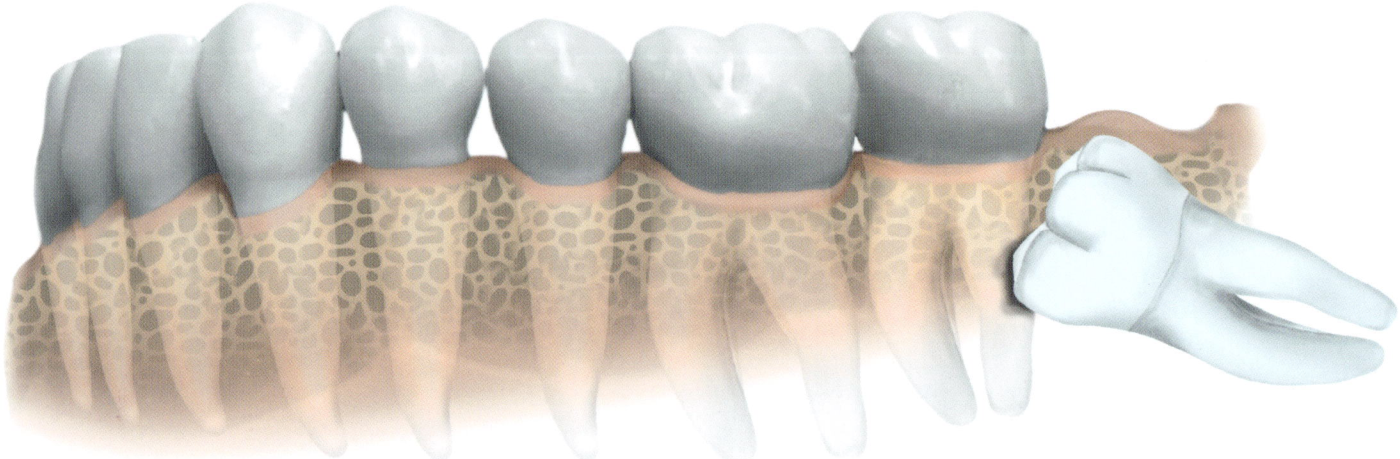

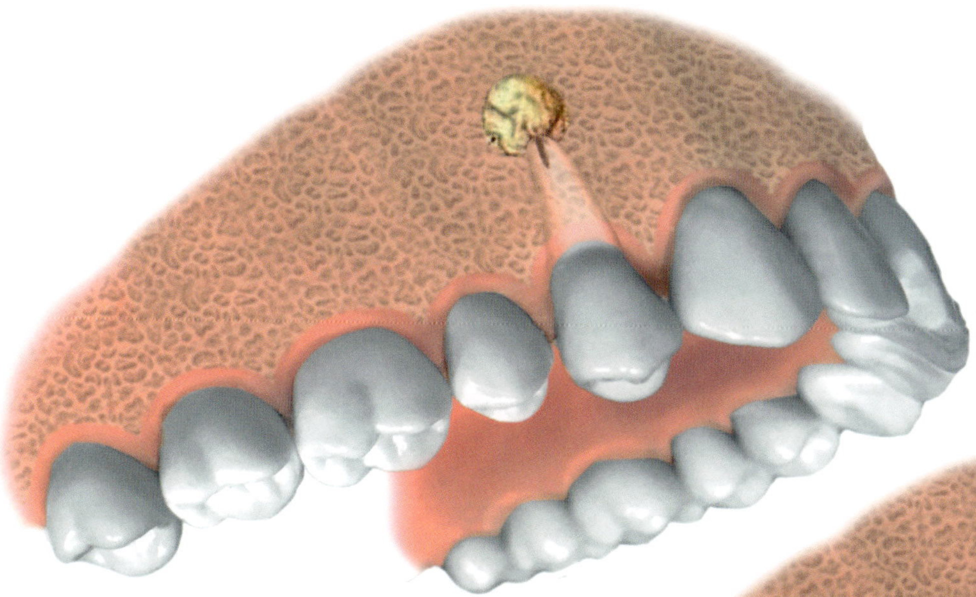

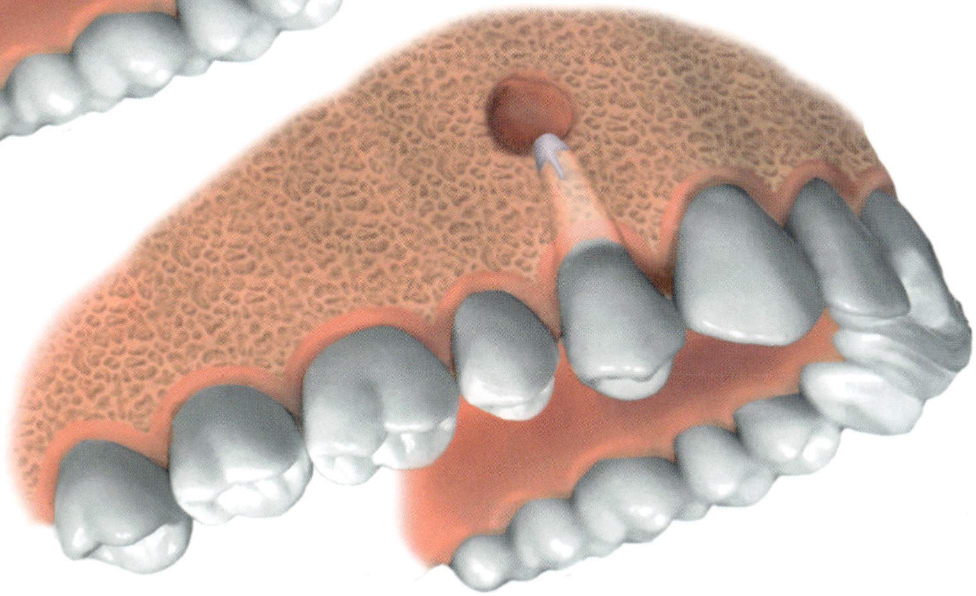

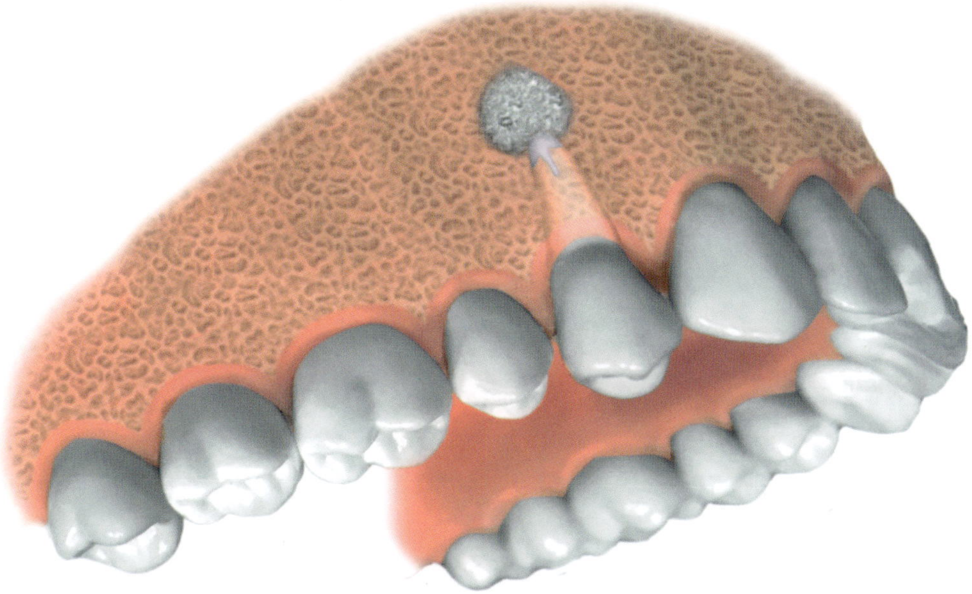

Surgery that has the same objective as endodontic therapy, but adopting a "retrograde" surgical approach by which the periapical area will be directly accessed; the granuloma will be removed and the most apical part of the tooth root will be removed.

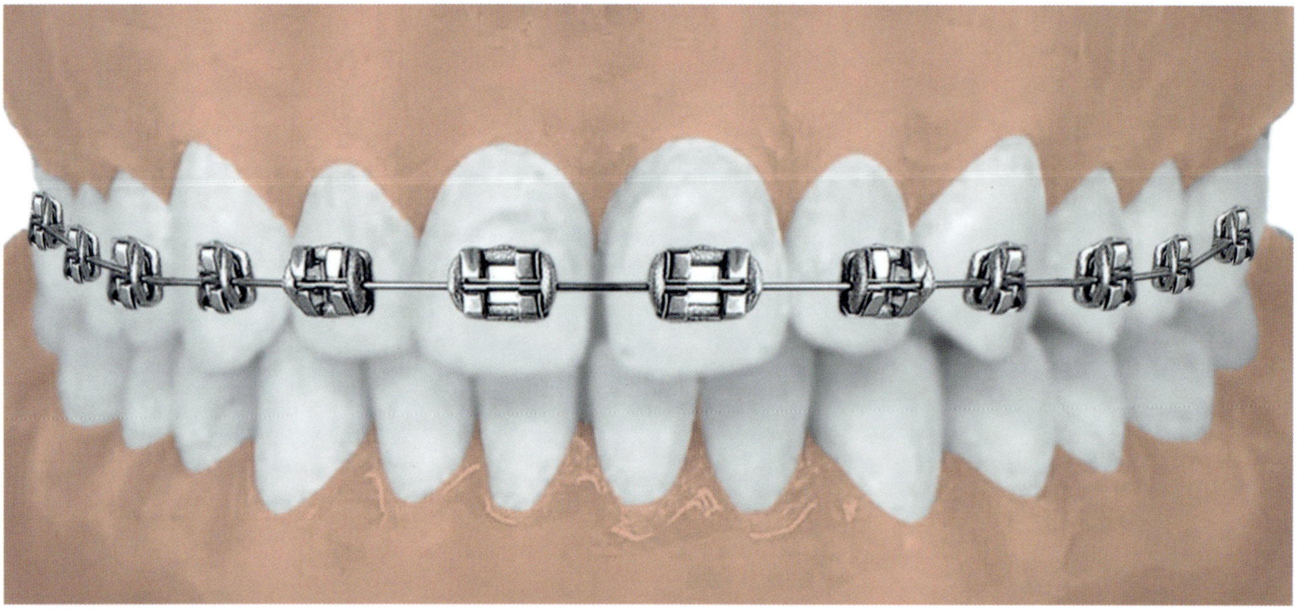

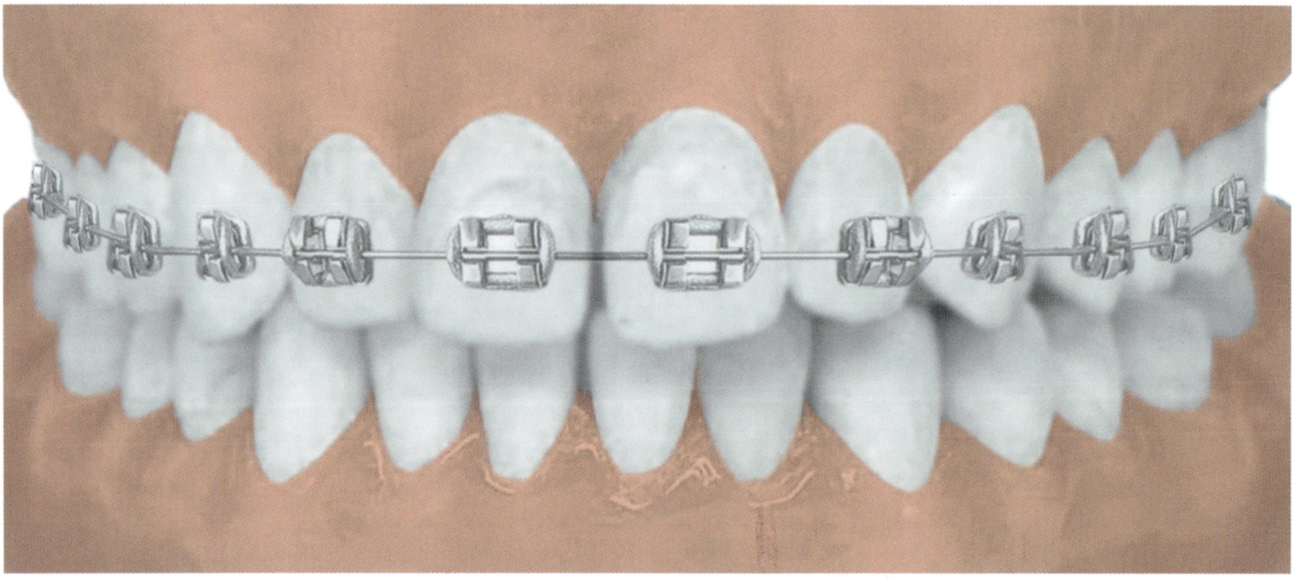

Above, classic multibrackets appliance used to correct dental disharmonies and misalignments. It consists of brackets, archwires and ligatures that act together to stimulate dental displacement.

Below, aesthetic variant of the multibracket appliances. The brackets here are made of ceramic while the wire is made more pleasing to the eye thanks to a coating that gives it a tooth-like color.

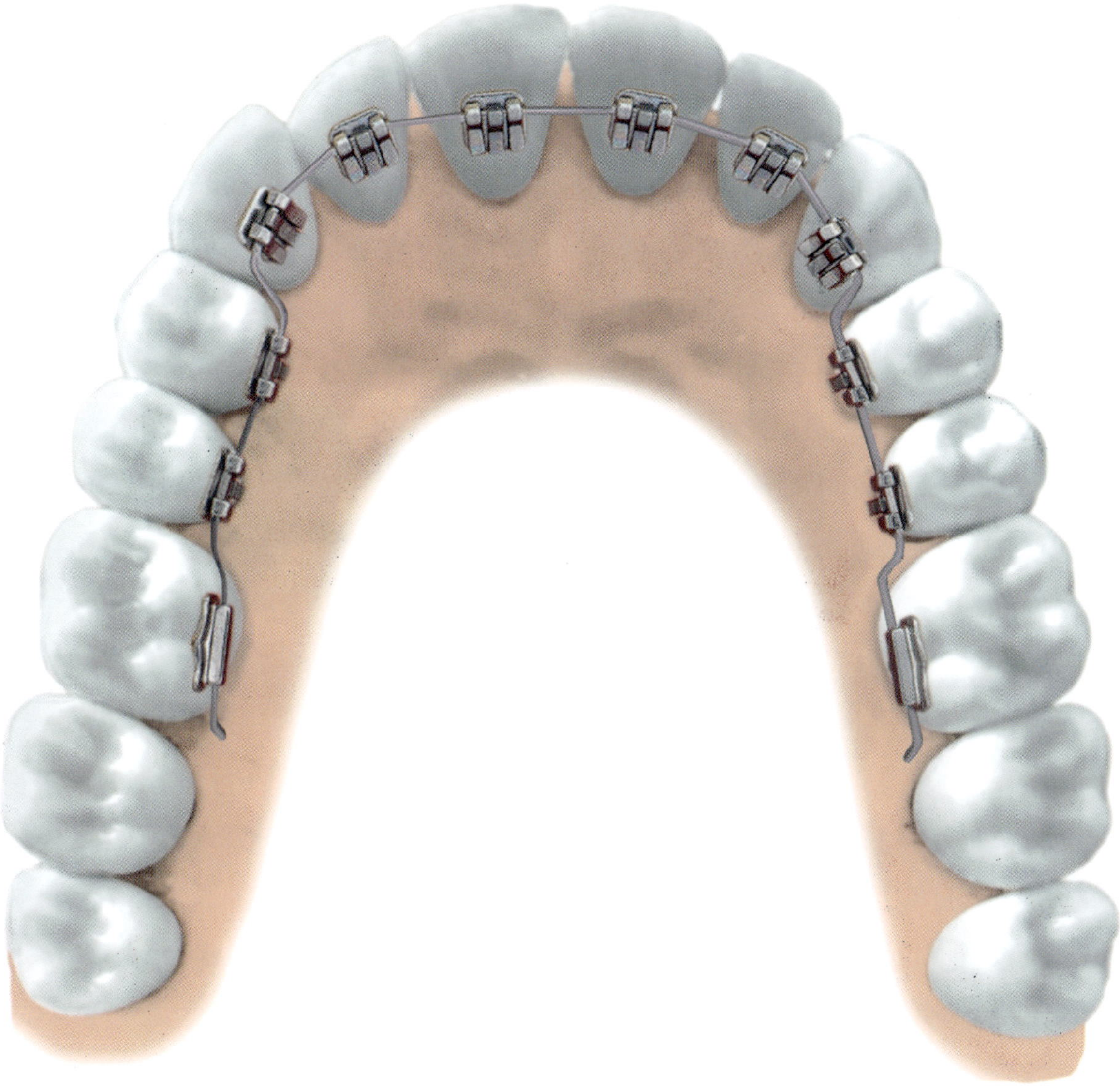

Lingual variant of the multibracket appliances. All the components are mounted on the side, whether upper or lower.

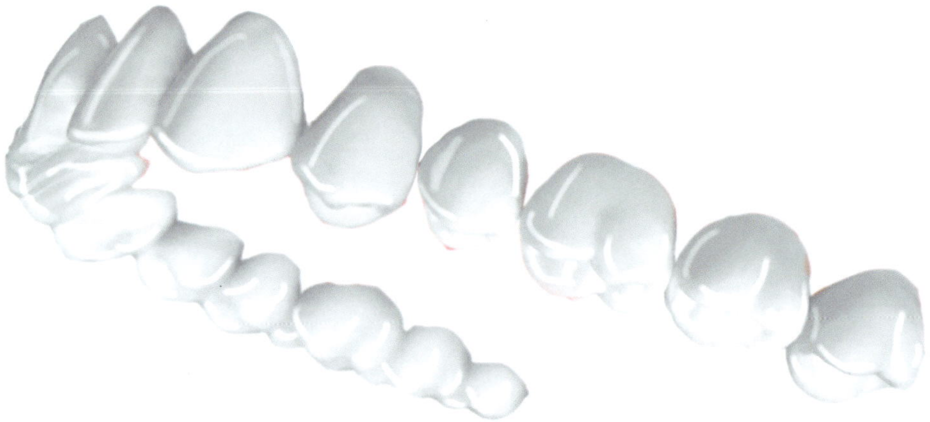

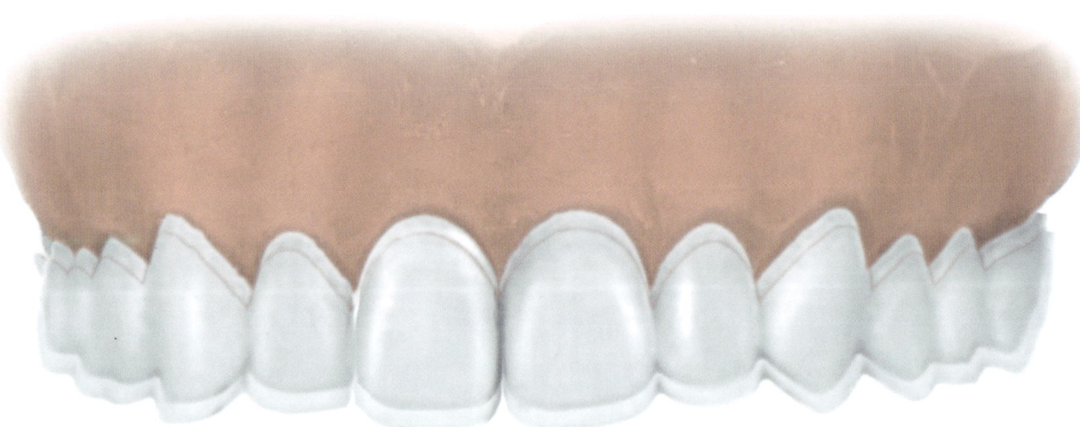

Invisible appliance.
It consists of several masks that will be progressively replaced allowing dental alignment to be achieved gradually.

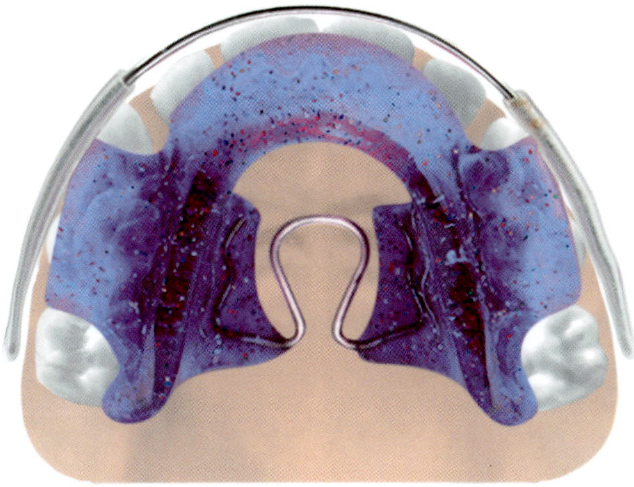

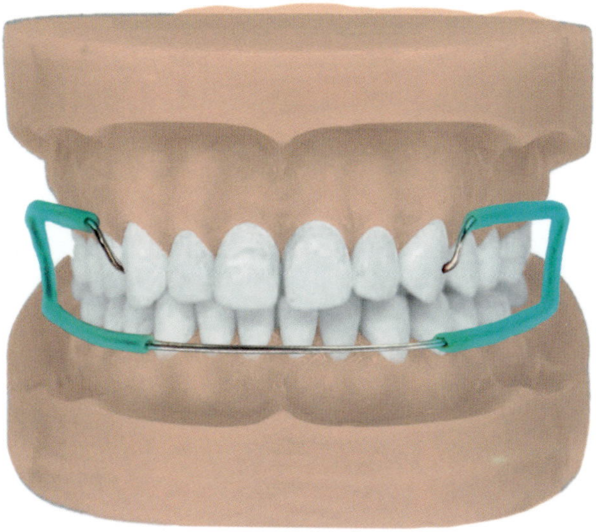

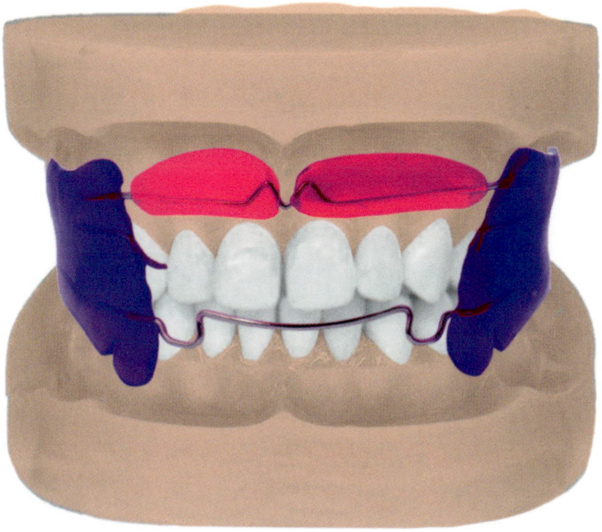

Mobile appliance to develop forces on the teeth or jaws.
They are aimed at harnessing muscle tone and modify the balance between the external and internal muscles of the arches, so as to favor tooth and jaw movement in the three dimensions of space.

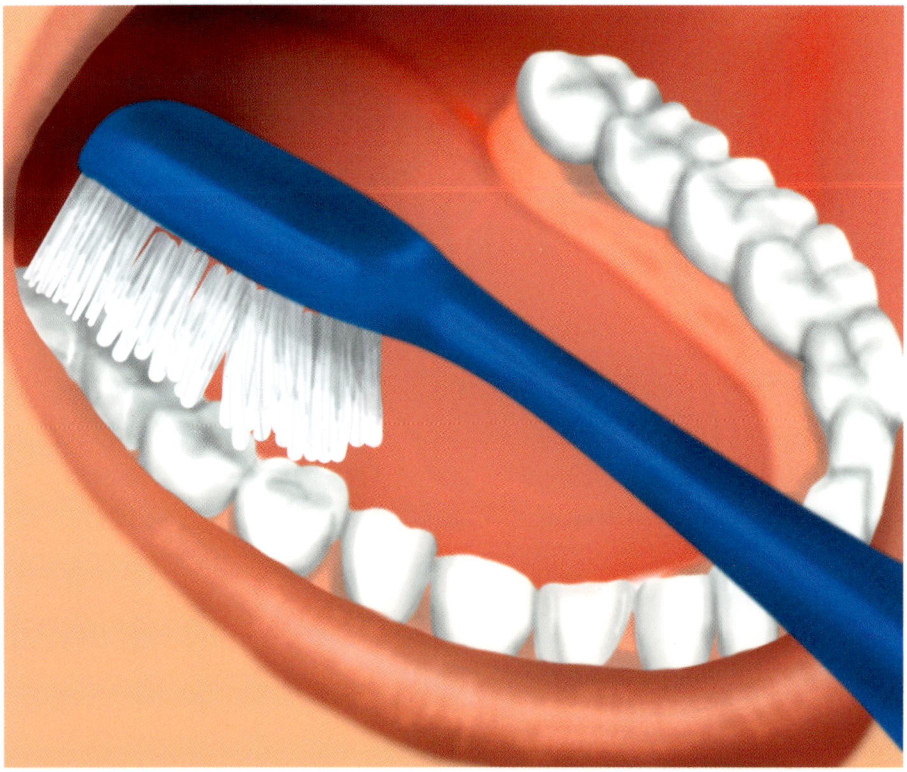

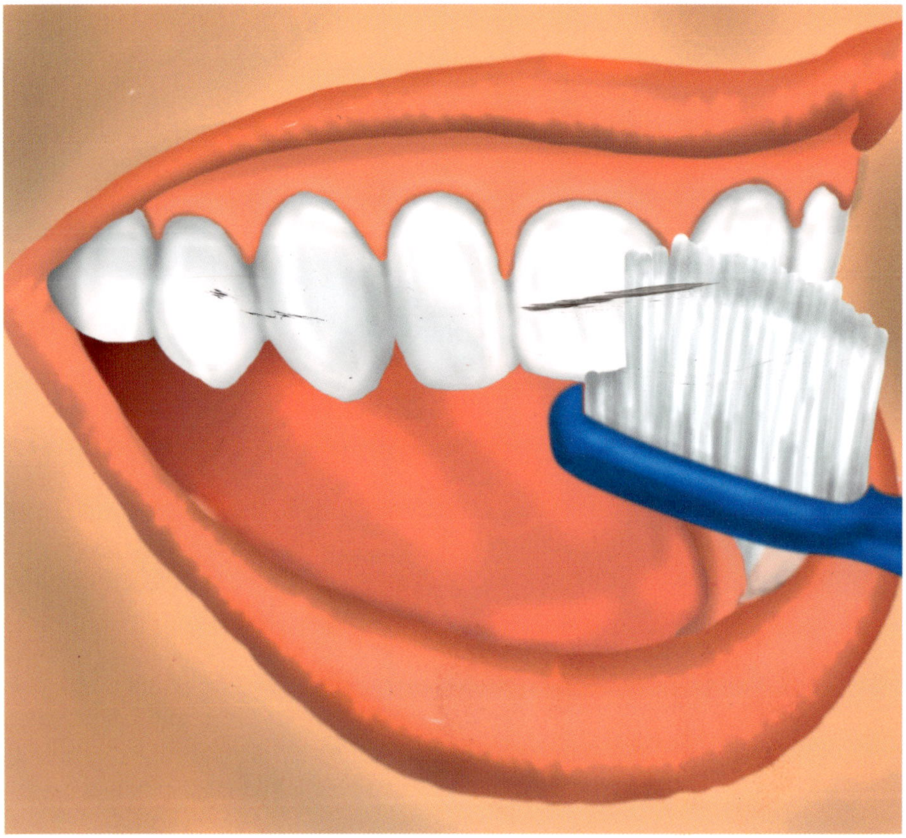

To make home oral hygiene maneuvers effective, it will be necessary to use the toothbrush correctly, making rotational movements along the entire arch in the apical-coronal direction, i.e., from the gingiva toward the teeth.

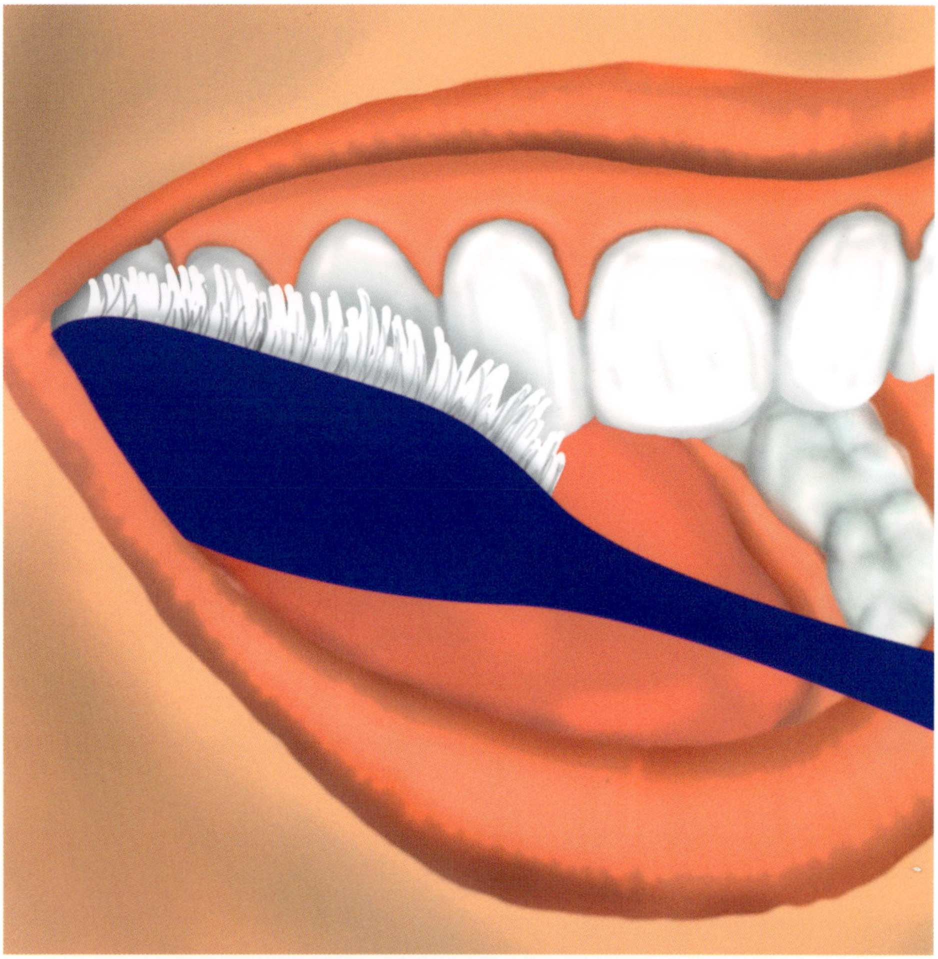

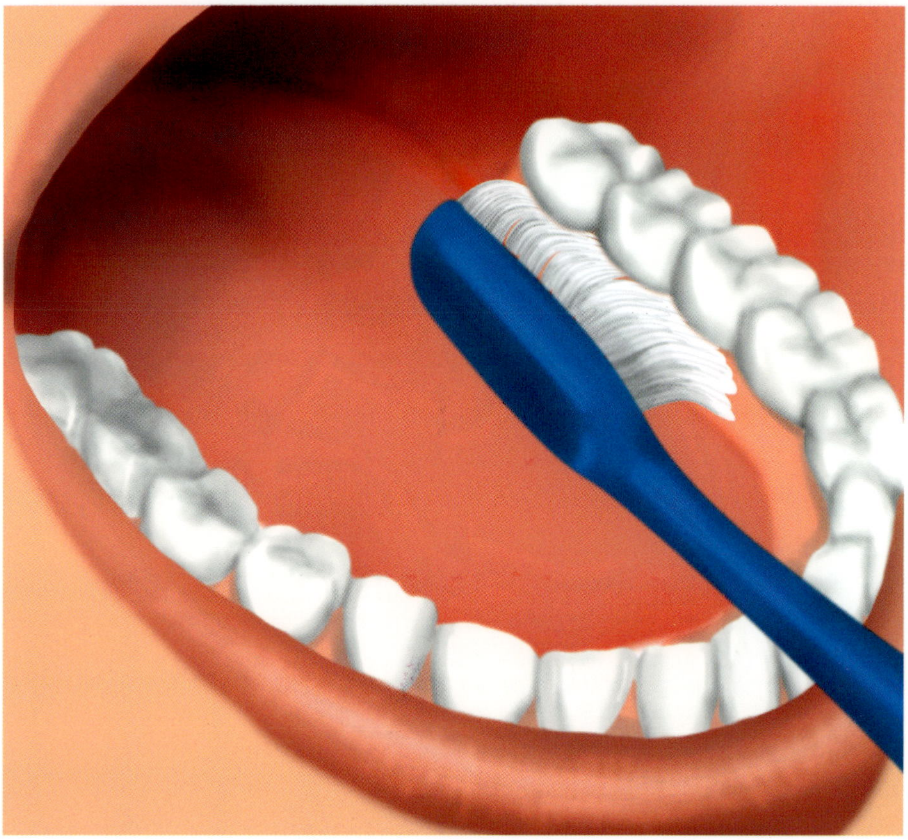

These rotations must also be performed internally in both arches. Finally, the toothbrush will have to be rubbed on the occlusal surfaces of the teeth, i.e., those deputed to chewing.

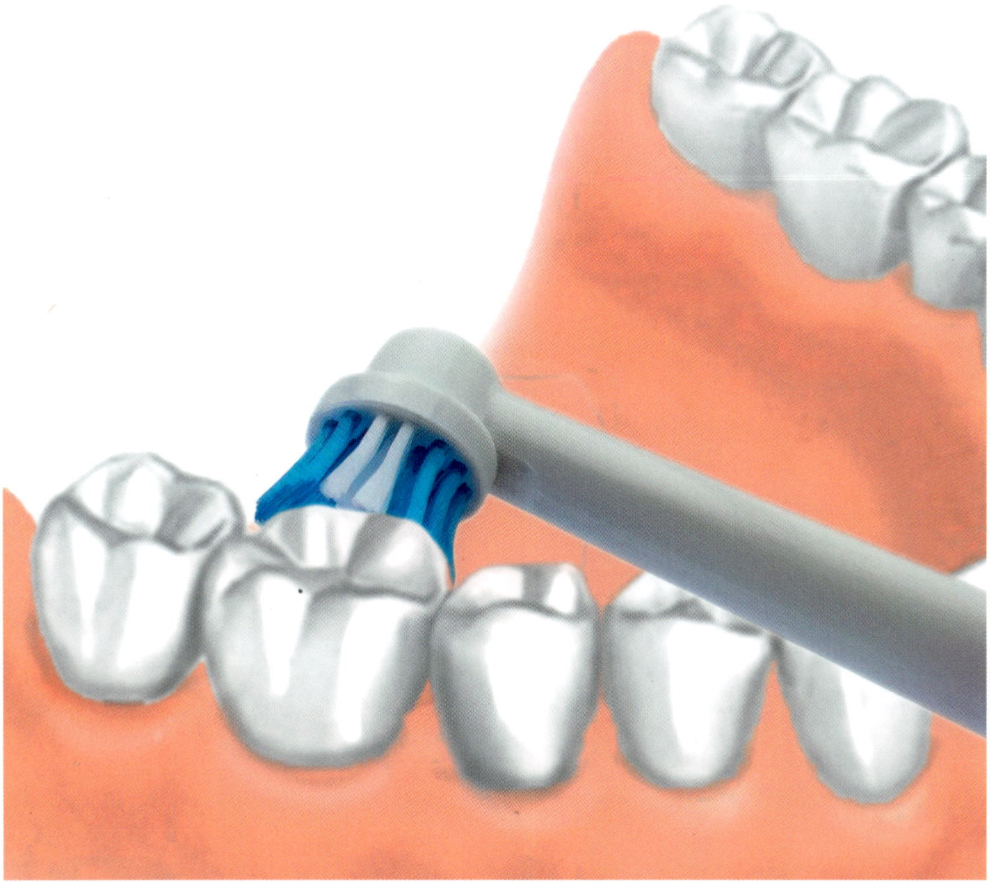

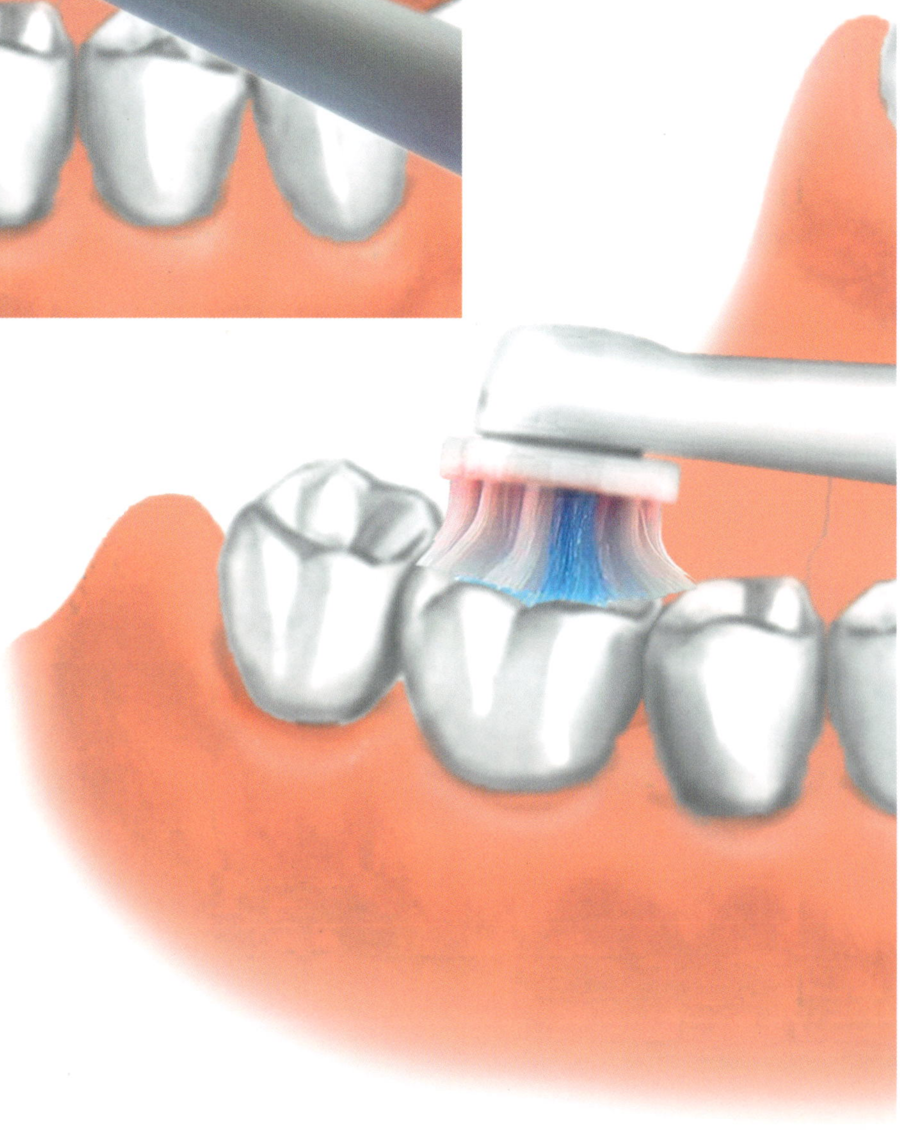

The electric variant of the toothbrush has a round head, similar in size to that of a tooth. Unlike the manual toothbrush, in this case the brush head is expected to remain stationary for 2-3 seconds on each dental surface: vestibular; lingual/palatal; occlusal.

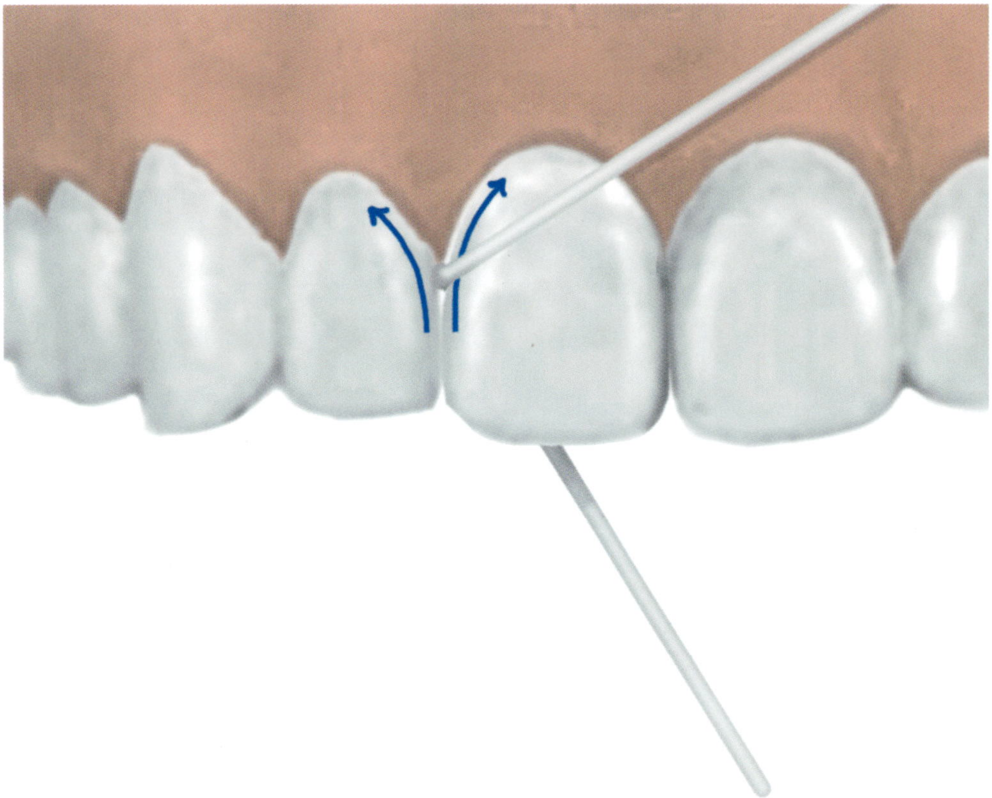

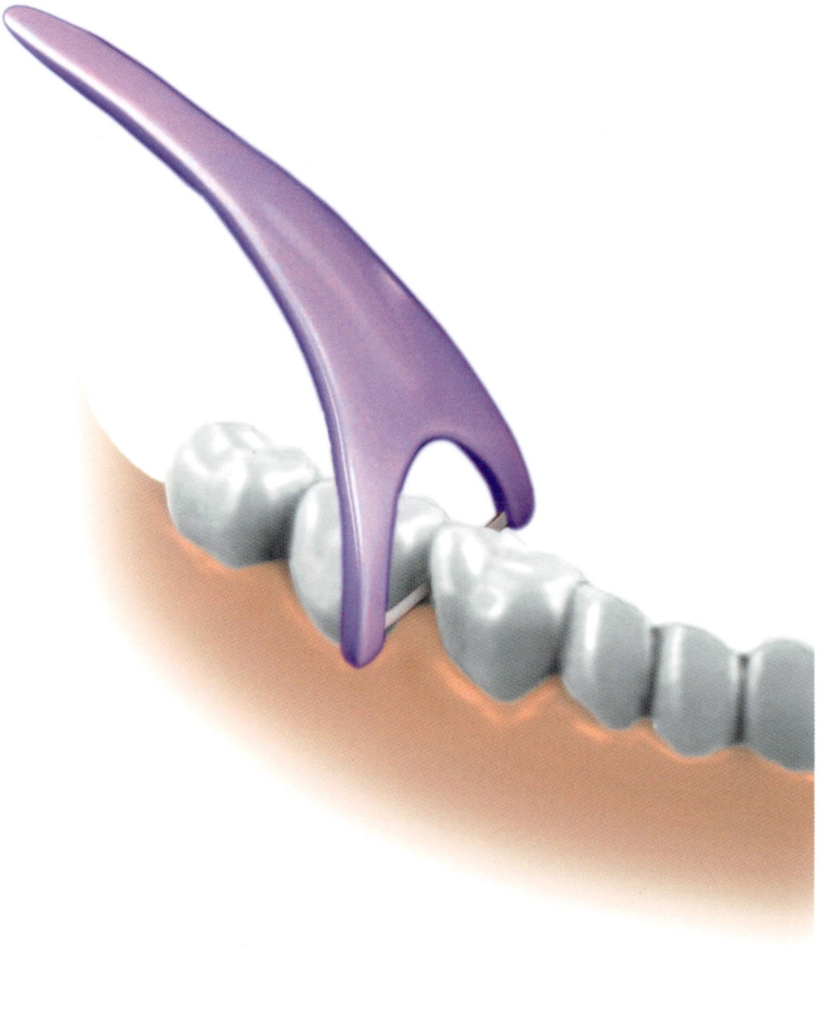

The correct use of dental floss involves inserting it below the contact point and then wrapping it around the tooth. In this way, the rubbing will be effective as it will help to accurately remove food residues between the tooth and the gingiva, as well as between tooth and tooth. The tension floss holder is a variant of using dental floss which, through an arch on which the dental floss is stretched, allows for more practical and immediate use.

INTERDENTAL TOOTHBRUSH

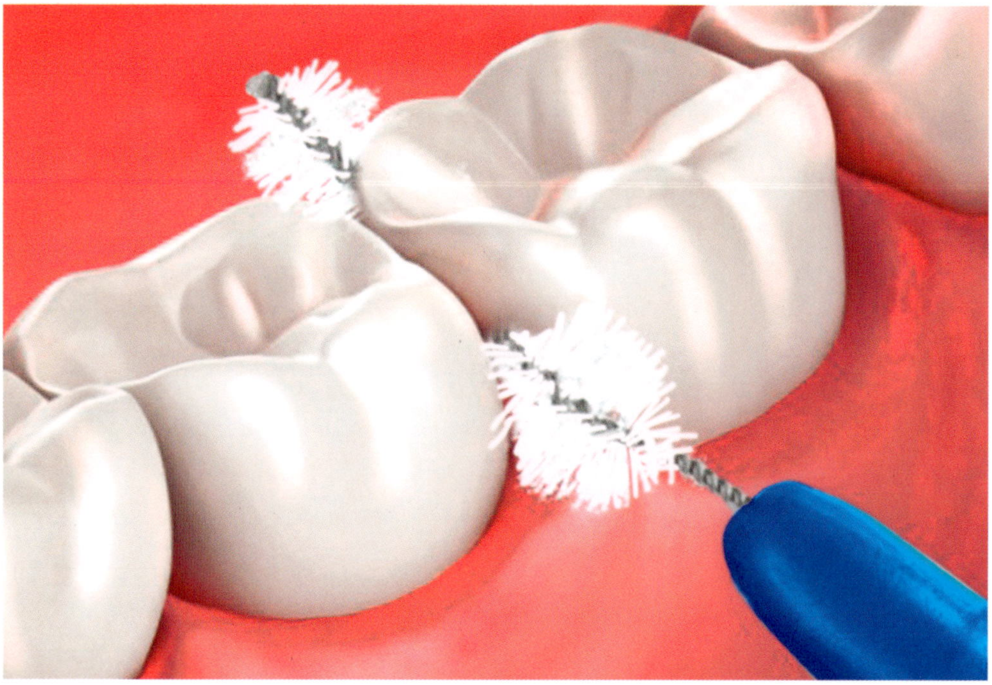

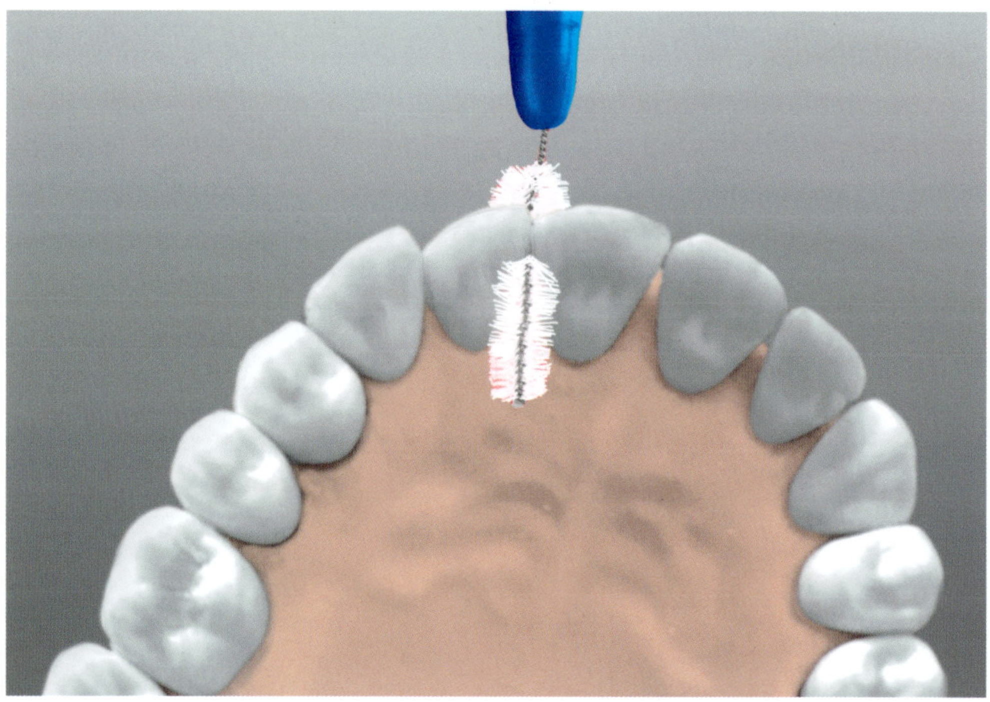

This tool is used in addition to dental floss, to remove food residues between one tooth and another, simultaneously massaging the interdental papilla.

CONSEQUENCE OF THE LOSS OF 46 WITH EXTRUSION OF 16 AND INCLINATION OF 45 AND 47

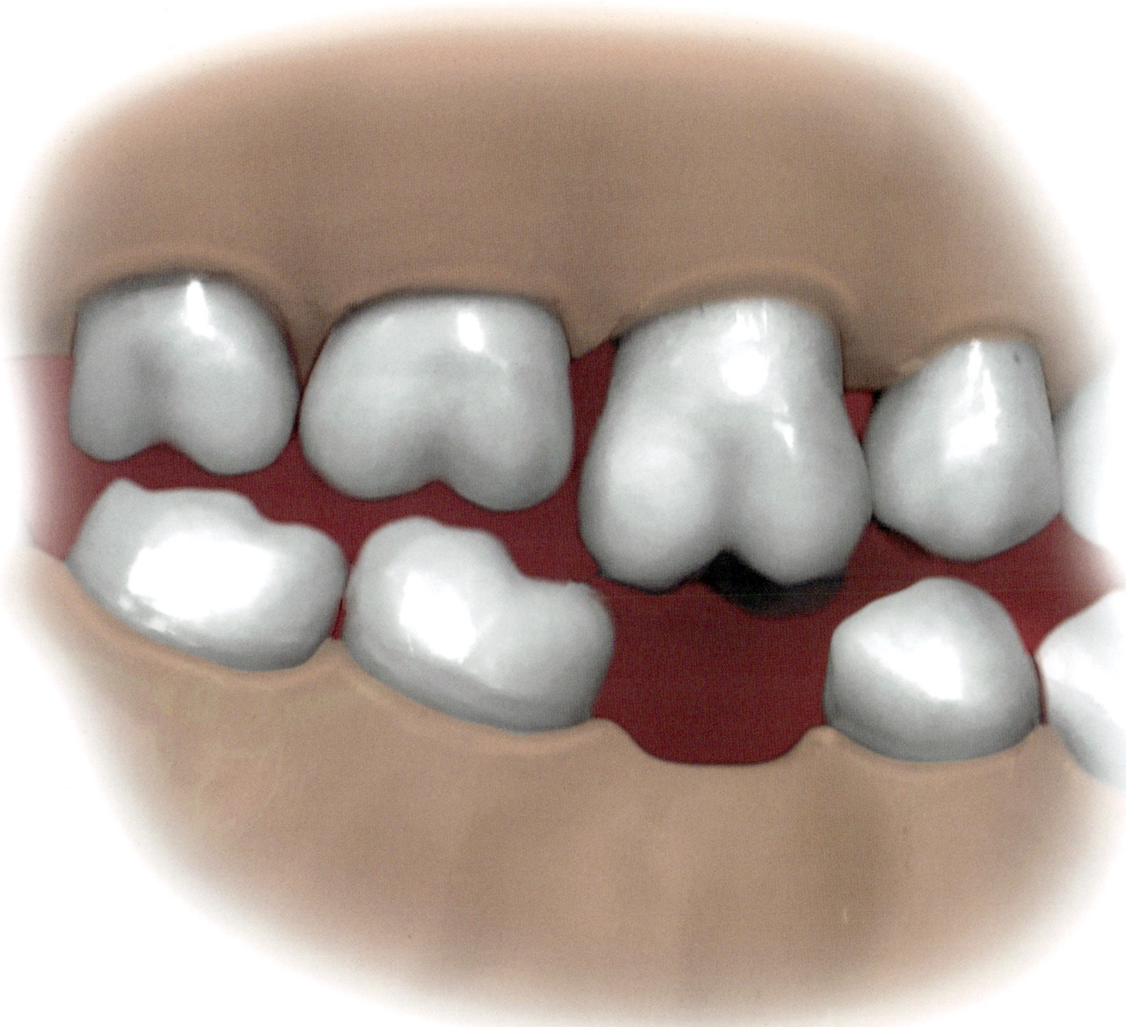

Following the loss of the lower first molar, the upper first molar will tend to extrude (descend), while the adjacent teeth will tend to tilt towards the edentulous gap.

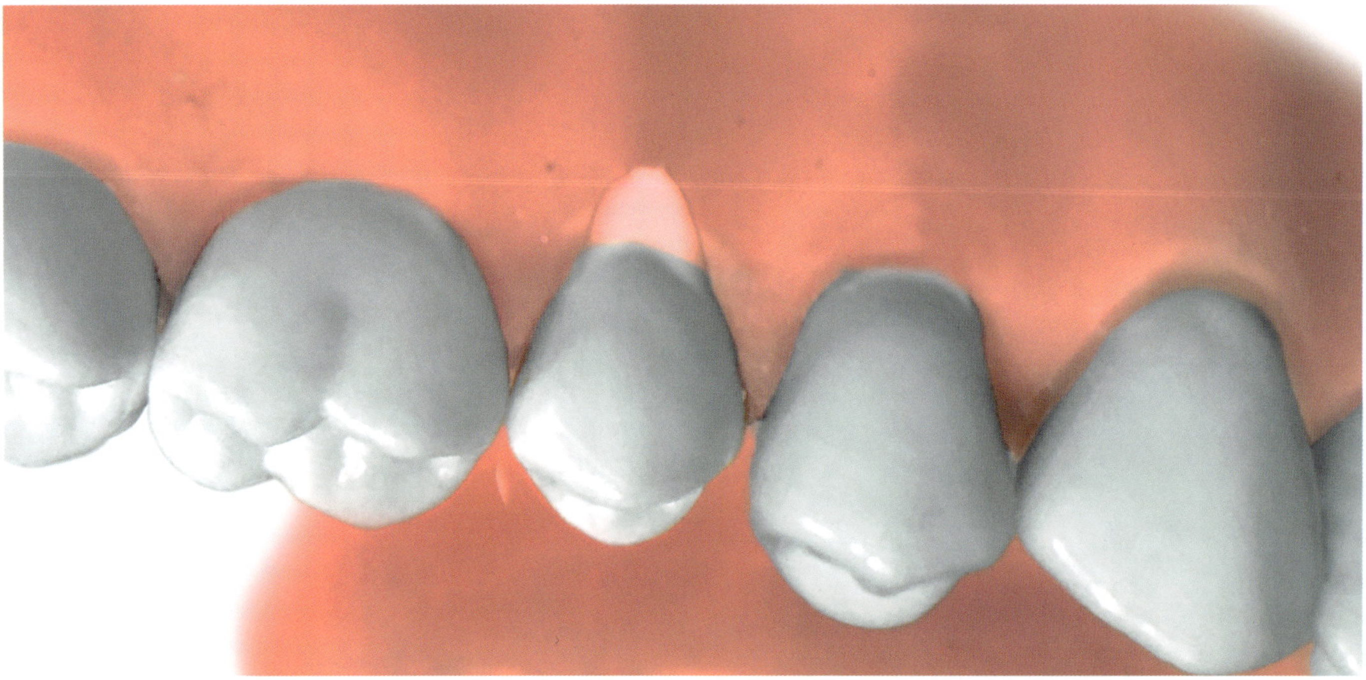

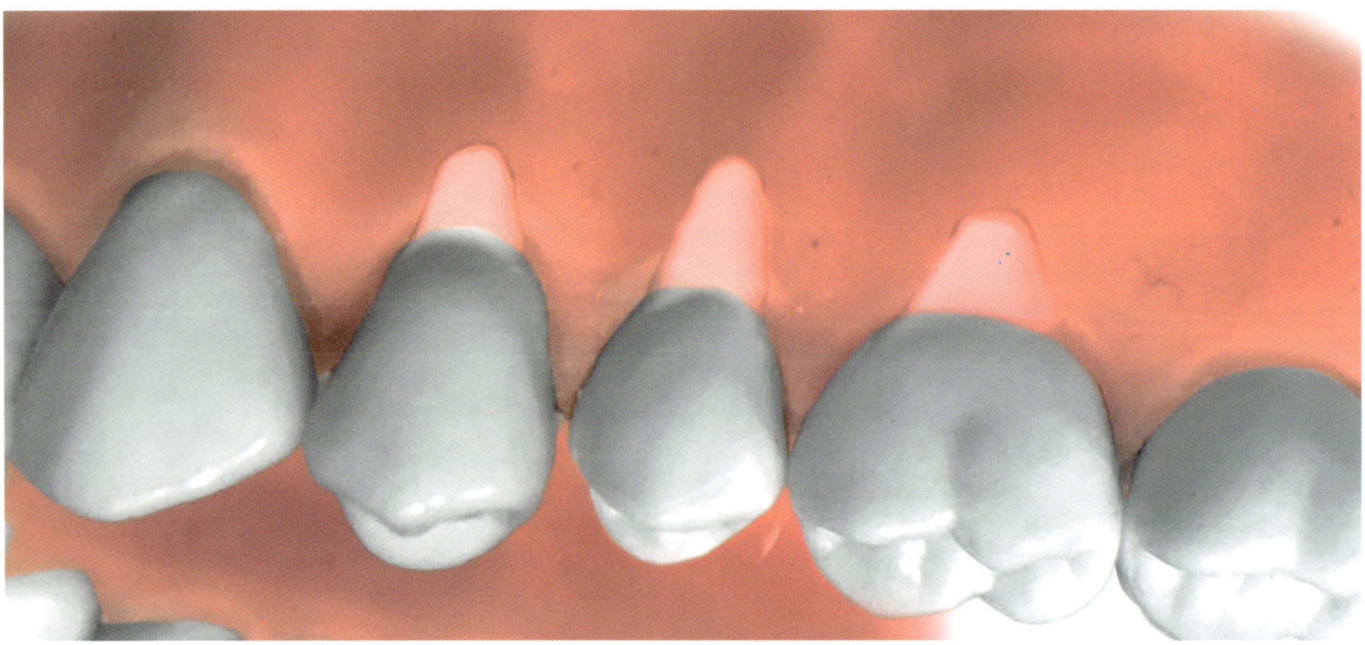

One of the most frequent causes of dentinal hypersensitivity is the exposure of portions of the root cement following gingival recession. This can be single or multiple.

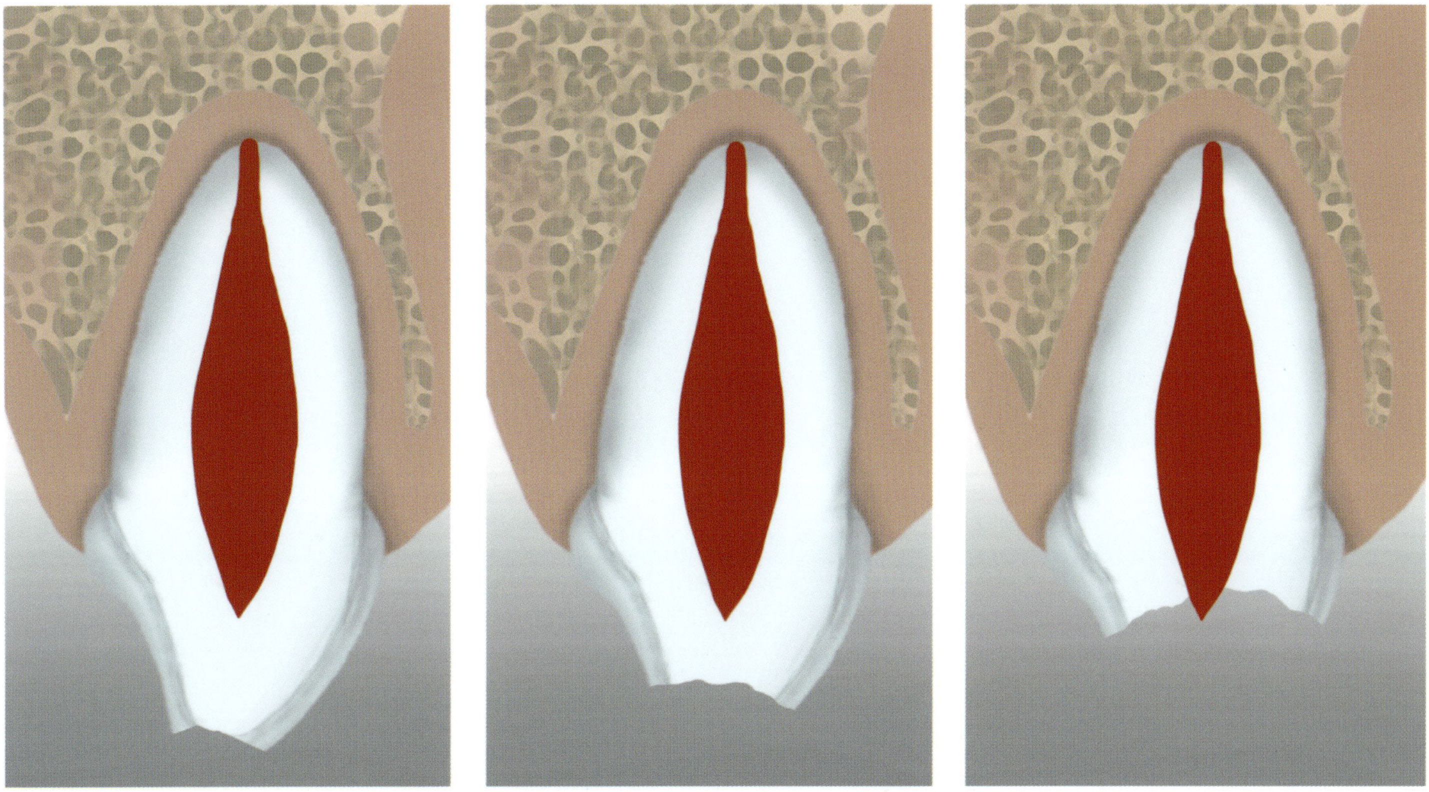

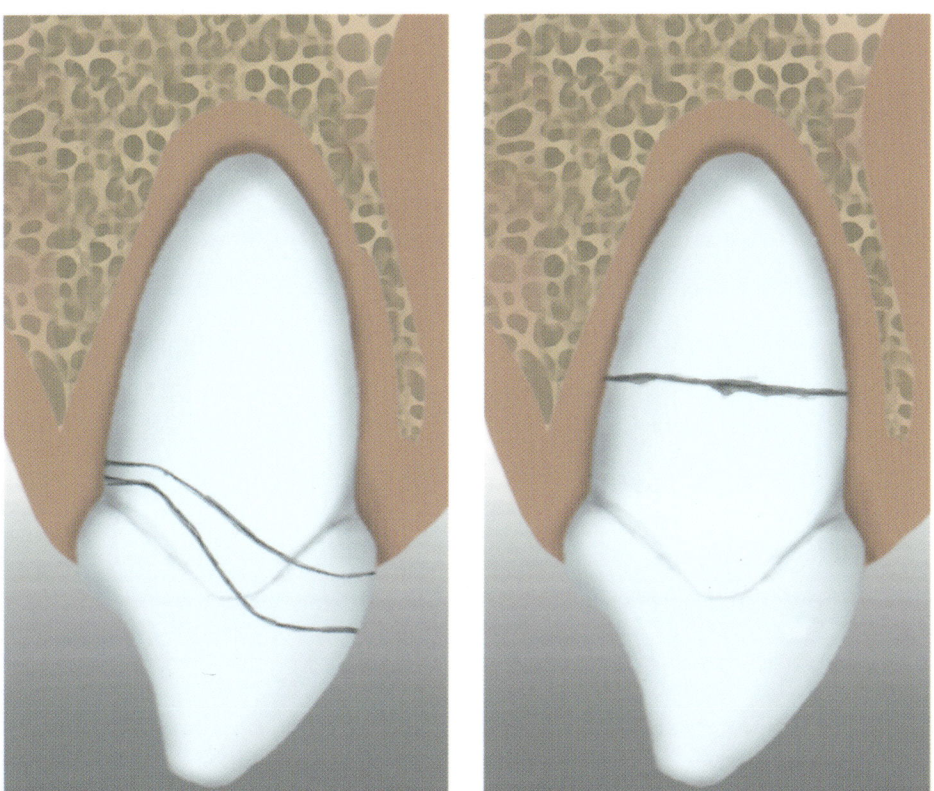

In order: coronal fracture; uncomplicated coronal fracture; complicated coronal fracture; uncomplicated or complicated crown-root fracture (see fracture line); root fracture.